T0144424

BASIC HEALTH PUBLICATIONS USER'S GUIDE

TO GARLIC

Learn How This Remarkable Food Can Reduce Your Risk of Heart Disease and Cancer.

DR. STEPHEN FULDER
with TINA SILVERMAN
JACK CHALLEM Series Editor

The information contained in this book is based upon the research and personal and professional experiences of the authors. It is not intended as a substitute for con sulting with your physician or other healthcare provider. Any attempt to diagnose and treat an illness should be done under the direction of a healthcare professional.

The publisher does not advocate the use of any particular healthcare protocol but believes the information in this book should be available to the public. The publisher and authors are not responsible for any adverse effects or consequences resulting from the use of the suggestions, preparations, or procedures discussed in this book. Should the reader have any questions concerning the appropriateness of any procedures or preparations mentioned, the authors and the publisher strongly suggest consulting a professional healthcare advisor.

Series Editor: Jack Challem
Editor: Susan Andrews
Typesetter: Gary A. Rosenberg
Series Cover Designer: Mike Stromberg

Basic Health Publications User's Guides are published by Basic Health Publications, Inc.

Copyright © 2005 by Dr. Stephen Fulder
ISBN: 978-1-59120-135-9 (Pbk.)
ISBN: 978-1-68162-853-0 (Hardcover)

CONTENTS

Introduction, 1

1. Garlic—The People's Panacea, 3

2. Reduce Cholesterol with Garlic, 12

3. Garlic and a Healthy Heart, 23

4. Garlic—The Detox Herb, 35

5. Garlic—The Natural Antibiotic, 42

6. The Essence of Garlic, 52

7. Garlic's History and Global Healing, 58

8. Garlic in Your Kitchen and Garden, 67

9. Garlic Supplements, 75

Conclusion, 85

Selected References, 86

Other Books and Resources, 88

Index, 89

INTRODUCTION

Garlic. The pungent, silky-smooth, creamy-white clove that adds abundant flavor and depth to the cuisines of the world is also one of the planet's most extraordinary natural medicines. Chopped, crushed, tossed into a sauce just before serving, or compressed into powder form in a capsule, garlic works wonders for your health.

If garlic were "invented" today in a chemical laboratory by a major drug manufacturer, this herb would be hailed as the miracle drug of the century. Imagine a medicine that can address so many health problems and has no dangerous side effects. A medicine that is cheap to buy and can even be grown in your own garden.

Sales of garlic supplements in the United States alone reach into the hundreds of millions of dollars every year. In Europe, where a centuries-old tradition of natural medicines remains strong, around 5 million people take garlic each day. Hundreds of studies are persuading doctors to take garlic seriously. Garlic's vital importance as a health aid is at last being recognized. Every few months, research groups are confirming that garlic is one of the best preventive remedies of all time. The beauty of this herb is that it works simultaneously on several levels. Studies have proved that garlic can lower cholesterol safely and easily. At the same time, they have shown that garlic can cause mild reductions in blood pressure. Its remarkable ability to thin the blood may help prevent clotting or thromboses in the blood vessels and reduce the risk of deadly or debilitating strokes. In short, garlic protects the heart and circulation. Used in small amounts, garlic is an excellent, natural way to cleanse the body of harmful chemicals, waste, and toxins. It is a wonderful all-round household cure for colds, chest and throat problems, mouth infections, Candida, and many other mild chronic infections.

This book will deal principally with the current research that has been carried out on garlic and how garlic can help to reduce the risk of heart disease. You'll learn what garlic is used for, how and why garlic works, and how you can use it to deal with specific health problems, such as high blood cholesterol. In the following pages, you'll learn how easy it is to incorporate garlic into your diet and health regimen. Many people hear about the healing properties of fresh garlic, but shy away from using it because of its sharp taste or the odorous breath it can cause. This guide will provide you with specific instructions on how to take fresh garlic without its social downside and how to buy the various garlic products currently available on the market. A grower's guide is included in Chapter 8, so that you can easily enjoy the pleasures of cultivating this health resource by yourself.

Finally, garlic is more than just a medicine. We'll discuss its fascinating place in history and its important place in the world's cuisine and dietary habits. A well-known saying expresses it all: *L'ail est sante. Mangez de l'ail.* "Garlic is health. Eat it." Enjoy!

CHAPTER 1

GARLIC— THE PEOPLE'S PANACEA

There is nothing new about garlic's use as a medicine. It is one of the oldest remedies known to humans and was used without interruption for a wide variety of ailments until a century ago. Only for a comparatively short period of time in human history, since the early 1900s, has garlic disappeared from common use as a medicine. Garlic, along with most herbs, was replaced by synthetic drugs. Now, however, garlic is being rediscovered. People are coming to realize that its benefits are highly relevant to some of the most widespread health problems of our time.

Mankind and garlic have had a long and passionate relationship as both a food and a medicine. Just as cultivated garlic has needed man to ensure its propagation, so man has needed garlic to guard his health, well-being, and vigor. This herb is part of our culture and human heritage. Its wide range of medicinal usage is backed by thousands of years of tradition. Because garlic can help alleviate a wide range of common health problems, it continues to be the number one household remedy for people all over the globe. Even in ancient times it was known as "The Peasant's Panacea," because simple country folk used garlic to cure themselves without having to rely on ex - pensive and sophisticated medicines.

Today, there are hundreds of research studies to support its healing powers. Scientific and medical journals, from the *Scientific American* to the *Lancet*, have published high-quality research on

Panacea
The name often given to a "cure-all" remedy that is thought to cure a wide range of different health problems.

garlic. Besides the bulbs themselves, you can find garlic products on the shelves of every health food store and pharmacy. Recently, it has been given as much prominence in the media as any new drug, and a lot more publicity than almost any other herbal remedy. Garlic has become one of the most popular and talked about natural remedies of all time. Let's see why.

Why Garlic Is Special

It is no wonder that throughout the ages garlic has become famous as a "Cure-All." Garlic offers a level of multiple protection to an extent that no single modern drug is able to provide. Yet it is a food that millions of people take in their diet daily throughout life without any ill effects. No wonder it has been praised for centuries as one of the main health aids known to humankind, a readily available and inexpensive preventive that should be in every household kitchen and medicine cabinet. Evidence of human's belief in garlic's curative powers was found in King Tutankhamen's Tomb and Aristotle recommended garlic as a soothing tonic (see Chapter 7 for a fascinating look at the history of garlic). No wonder that it is described in history as "The People's Panacea."

Garlic wins the Triple Crown in the natural medicinal herb competition. It finishes first because it can successfully address three major aspects of health: (1) Garlic is the key to a healthy heart, (2) it is instrumental in cancer prevention, and (3) it is a powerful way to treat a wide variety of common infections. We will briefly review these uses here and then explore them more fully in later chapters.

Garlic and a Healthy Heart

The fact that heart disease is now the major cause

of death in developed nations has led to an intense scientific search for natural remedies that will help the heart harmlessly. Doctors, too, have shown increasing interest. Because pharmaceutical drugs that are available to reduce the amount of cholesterol in the blood often have side effects, doctors have been reluctant to prescribe them too widely. Understandably, most doctors are reluctant to turn most of the population into patients.

The natural solution is garlic. From the ancient knowledge of Indian and Eastern medicine we know that garlic removes fats from the blood and protects the heart. Traditional herb books, professional herbalists, and naturopathic doctors always recommend garlic to those with circulatory problems who are at risk of heart attack. They state that garlic opens the blood vessels and thins the blood, and a considerable body of modern, scientific research has confirmed this traditional picture.

Here's how it works: An excess of fat and cholesterol is one of the major causes of the buildup of arterial blockages. Arterial blockage is the cause of circulatory disease, heart attacks, and strokes. As we mentioned earlier, garlic lowers the levels of fat and cholesterol in the blood, and it does this as well as, or even better than, the modern drugs now used for this purpose.

Studies at some major research centers in the United States, such as the Department of Biochemistry at the George Washington University School of Medicine in Washington, D.C., have confirmed that garlic does indeed thin the blood by reducing its tendency to clot inside the blood vessels. It does this at quite a low dose—less than a clove a day can make a difference that is clearly measurable in the laboratory. Since clots can suddenly block blood vessels, they, too, are one of the main, immediate causes of heart attacks, angina, and strokes. Garlic may be able to directly reduce the risks of these health catastrophes.

in German pharmacies. Unlike in other countries, garlic is not frequently used in the diet in Germany, where many people prefer to take garlic in the form of tablets and capsules. Garlic's popularity as a medicine in Germany is indeed astonishing—nearly 1 million Germans now regularly take garlic products, primarily to prevent heart disease.

In Japan, too, garlic preparations have been accepted by the Health Ministry as means of reducing blood pressure. Garlic also appears in the official drug guides of such countries as Spain and Switzerland.

Similar developments are taking place in the United Kingdom. According to a recent poll, 10 percent of the British population has used garlic or garlic products for medicinal purposes. Although the British medical authorities have not yet accepted garlic's effectiveness as a remedy for circulatory problems, they have acknowledged its other main popular use, that of combating infections. The United Kingdom's Ministry of Health permits garlic product manufacturers to claim that garlic is "an herbal remedy traditionally used for the treatment of the symptoms of common cold and cough" and "an herbal remedy traditionally used for temporary relief of symptoms of rhinitis and catarrh." Although theirs is a cautious, conservative approach, it does show that the United Kingdom's leading drug experts recognize garlic's medicinal potential. Garlic is clearly a highly popular natural medicine, widely accepted throughout the world and steadily becoming acknowledged by the medical authorities.

Above all, garlic is safe. Millions of people have included garlic in their daily diet throughout their lives without any ill effects, and there is no evidence in the scientific literature of any adverse effects from taking garlic in normal doses as a medicine. No wonder it has been praised for thousands of years as a primary health aid. Garlic is a readily available and inexpensive preventive that should be in every household kitchen and medicine cabinet.

Medicines Can Also Be Foods

The garlic plant that is used as a medicine is the same one that is used throughout the world for flavoring. As a food, garlic adds richness, taste, aroma, and nutrients to salads, meat, fish, and vegetable dishes. In Asian, Chinese, Middle Eastern, Mediterranean, and European cuisine, garlic is often a central ingredient and appears in thousands of delicious recipes.

The rising popularity of garlic as a health supplement led to a cartoon in the *New York Times*, showing a bemused consumer reading a "Prescription Only" sign posted over the vegetable aisle at the supermarket. To anyone who has lived within the rich cultural traditions of countries like India and China, there is little doubt that foods can be medicines, and medicines can be foods.

There is a veritable pharmacy on your kitchen shelves and in your refrigerator. You may already know that fiber is great for digestive problems. Oats, barley, and green tea can aid in lowering cholesterol. Vegetables rich in beta-carotene can help prevent cancer. Fish oil and olive oil help prevent heart disease. Clove oil works as a pain-killer for toothaches. Brew a tea from thyme to ease the pain of a sore throat. The list goes on and on. In an article published in 2000 in the medical journal *Chest*, Dr. Stephen Rennard of the University of Nebraska Medical Center, gave scientific evidence that validates what our grandmothers knew all along—when you have a cold, a hot bowl of chicken soup has remarkable healing and soothing powers.

Medicinal Foods
Spices, herbs, and plants that have a therapeutic as well as a nutritional effect on our bodies.

"Let your food be your medicine," said Hippocrates, the father of medicine, who compiled a list of over 400 herbs and their uses. Herbs, spices, and other nutritional substances are the oldest form of medicine known to man. In some societies the knowledge of foods' medicinal power is vast.

Culinary Herbs and Spices

Herbs are usually aromatic tasty leaves that are used dried or fresh. Spices are dried seeds or barks, normally grown in hot climates.

Acquiring this knowledge, handed down through the generations, can take years. In India, in traditional families, the mother designs the daily menu to include those foods, vegetables, and spices that are most suitable for the place, the season, and the weather. She then cooks, using ingredients that treat the special vulnerabilities or health problems of the family members.

Spices are on the borderline between food and medicine. It may be hard to imagine the dry, old, bottled powders at the back of the kitchen cupboards as medicines. However, consider for a moment the bombshell to the body locked up in a few grains of cayenne pepper. How about the anesthetic effect of chewing cloves for a sore tooth, or the miraculous way a cup of strong sage tea will clear up a cold, and one of thyme tea, a sore throat. If you have experienced the effect of anise or fennel seeds on an upset stomach, or how a piece of ginger can alleviate morning sickness, you know something of the power of medicinal foods.

Culinary Herbs Are Effective and Reliable Remedies

As remedies, culinary herbs such as garlic have some distinct advantages over modern drugs. First and foremost, they are extremely safe. Second, they are cheap and readily available, without a doctor's prescription, all over the world. Third, culinary herbs and spices can be effective for conditions for which modern drugs are too strong and unnecessary. You can skip the expense and the time in visiting your doctor when your kitchen holds the answer for many mild common health problems, from indigestion to headaches. Fourth, medicinal foods can often be used to strengthen your resistance to disease. Apart from vaccines, most modern drugs only treat disease; they are not preventives.

Finally, herbs and spices do provide important nutritional benefits, because they contain vitamins and minerals. Best of all, they add great taste to your diet. Herbs and spices, especially garlic, enhance the pleasure of eating. Why depend on medical professionals when you can use a wide range of tasty herbs and spices as part of your self-care health regimen?

CHAPTER 2

REDUCE CHOLESTEROL WITH GARLIC

One of the great challenges in the field of health care is the fight to control the diseases of the heart and circulation. Because heart disease claims more lives every day than any other single cause, it is crucial that we search for ways to prevent this modern plague from growing. Every week, newspaper and magazine articles tell us about new drugs now being offered on the market that can reduce our chances of getting heart disease; however, each drug's benefits may be accompanied by side effects. Is there a natural way to reduce the risk? Must we rely on a pharmaceutical solution alone?

In this chapter we will focus on cholesterol, explaining what it is and how it contributes to heart disease. You will learn how to incorporate garlic into a wellness program designed to prevent or treat heart disease. We'll look at the effectiveness of garlic in reducing cholesterol, and how much garlic you need to reach your goal of a healthy heart. You'll find out how long garlic takes to work and how it can benefit you, even if your cholesterol is not particularly high.

Defining Raised Cholesterol

Cholesterol has nearly become a dirty word in today's world. Mention cholesterol and most people react with a sense of dread. But the truth is that the body needs cholesterol. This soft, waxy substance is used to build cell membranes and create hormones such as estrogen and testosterone. Cholesterol is made in the liver and our bodies can produce all the cholesterol we need.

However, when we are under continuous stress, the liver produces extra choles- terol to create the hormones needed to cope with excess emotional and psychological pressure. When our bodies create more cholesterol than we need, we face the dan- gers of heart disease.

Cholesterol
A soft, waxy sub - stance present in all parts of the body. Made in the liver and obtained from animal fats, it is essential for normal body functions in- cluding hormone production.

Additional cholesterol arrives with our food. In fact, the amount of cholesterol in the blood depends on several factors, which include:

1. The consumption of so-called saturated fats (the fat found in all animal and dairy prod- ucts), which encourages the liver to make more cholesterol

2. The cholesterol in our diet

3. Inadequate physical fitness (a major culprit in cholesterol buildup)

4. Stress (after a professional car race, a driver's blood serum—the blood with the red blood cells removed—appears milky, because it con- tains excess cholesterol)

5. Obesity (obesity is generally defined as a weight that is 20 percent above the standard for age and height)

6. Diabetes

7. Lack of dietary fiber (a diet with too much processed food)

8. Heredity (some people have a natural tenden- cy to higher levels of cholesterol)

The level of cholesterol in the blood is directly linked to heart attack risk. In the 1960s, high cholesterol was first recognized as a major risk factor for heart disease. But it wasn't until the 1980s, when testing cholesterol levels became more common, that health experts became concerned.

The World Health Organization has looked at worldwide cholesterol levels and has stated that, for cardiac health, the cholesterol level should be at a maximum of 200 milligrams (one-fifth gram) per 100 milliliters (1 deciliter) of blood. The U.S. National Institutes of Health agrees. At these target numbers, 105 million Americans have a total cholesterol level of 200 milligrams per deciliter or higher, a level at which cardiovascular risk begins to rise.

The Problem with Cholesterol

A blood level of cholesterol within the normal range is necessary for good health. The problem is that if there is excess cholesterol, it accumulates along the artery walls and is deposited as fatty lumps, decreasing blood flow, and eventually—if left untreated—completely blocking the blood vessels. When the arteries that feed the heart and brain get blocked the result is a heart attack or stroke.

An enormous number of scientific studies and statistics have supported the link between high cholesterol and heart disease. For example, animals fed a diet rich in cholesterol suffer from heart disease, while animals fed an ordinary diet do not. A fascinating study compared two different human populations, men living in East Finland and men living in Japan. The males of East Finland had the highest level of blood cholesterol in the world, averaging 260 milligrams of cholesterol to every 100 milliliters of blood. The Japanese men, on the other hand, had an average of 160 milligrams of cholesterol to every 100 milliliters of blood. And the heart attack level in East Finland was fourteen times greater than that in Japan!

A 10 percent reduction in cholesterol reduces the incidence of heart disease by 20 percent. In America, the average blood cholesterol level has declined 15 milligrams per 100 milliliters of blood in the past thirty years. This reduction can be attributed to dietary changes and increased involvement in fitness-oriented activities. Heart attacks have been reduced by as much as a third during that time, and the average life span has increased by three years. These are impressive figures indeed, and point to the connection between cholesterol levels and heart disease.

"Good" and "Bad" Cholesterol

To understand the workings of cholesterol in our bodies, it is important to take a brief look at exactly how cholesterol works. Cholesterol does not simply float around in oily drops in your blood. It is packaged inside little bags of protein called lipoproteins, which help it to dissolve in the blood. There are two main types of cholesterol/protein bags: LDL (low-density lipoprotein) and HDL (high-density lipoprotein).

LDL is considered the "bad" form of cholesterol, since it is the one taken up by the arteries to create fatty lumps. HDL, on the other hand, is called the "good" cholesterol because it may actually provide a protection against heart attacks. HDL seems to act as a kind of housecleaner, collecting the cholesterol from the walls of the arteries and returning it to the circulation.

It has now been found that people with high levels of HDL are protected from heart disease even if their overall cholesterol is high. In the now famous Framingham study, the risk of heart attack was 70 percent higher in those men with HDL less than 52 milligrams per 100 milliliters, compared to those with more HDL. In women it seemed to make even more of a difference. The women in the study whose HDL was less than 46 milligrams per 100 milliliters were six times more likely to have a heart attack than those with HDL levels above 67 milligrams per 100 milliliters. That is why, the HDL/LDL ratio is very often used as a measure of cardiovascular risk. The higher the ratio of HDL in the blood, the better the person's chances for avoiding heart disease.

Do I Have a Cholesterol Problem?

In May 2001, the U.S. National Institutes of Health (NIH) issued aggressive new cholesterol guidelines, suggesting that LDLs should be around 130 milligrams per 100 milliliters. Unfortunately, two-thirds of the adult population of modern, industrial countries have cholesterol levels well above this figure, and suffer from a great deal of heart disease.

It is a wise precaution to go to your family doctor for a cholesterol test. If your cholesterol is below 200 milligrams per 100 milliliters, it is "normal," that is, usual in our society. A level that falls within 200–270 milligrams per 100 milliliters should be taken as a warning sign to take better care of your circulation, and discuss the issue with your health professional. A level above 270 milligrams per 100 milliliters should be taken more seriously.

Garlic Significantly Reduces Cholesterol

With the relationship between high cholesterol levels and heart disease firmly established, it's time to discuss garlic's role in this equation. And, simply put, garlic is unparalleled as a means to lower the cholesterol levels in our blood.

In fact, as I've noted, garlic is rapidly becoming accepted as a safe cholesterol-lowering remedy within the conventional medical community. It has been the subject of a great deal of scientific and clinical research. More than thirty clinical studies from research centers all over the world have shown that garlic, at a dose of only one to two cloves per day, will lower cholesterol by about 15 percent. This decrease is enough to reduce the risk of a heart attack by 30 percent!

A typical study carried out by Professor F. H. Mader and his colleagues at several clinics in Germany, was published in 1990 in the journal *Drug Research*. The researchers gave garlic tablets at a relatively low dose, equivalent to less than one clove a day, to 261 people with raised blood cholesterol. Over a sixteen-week period there was an average drop in cholesterol of more than 10 percent. Those taking a placebo remained the same. None of the garlic-takers suffered any negative side effects, and few noticed the odor.

Several research teams have carried out a "meta-analysis," that is, a statistical summary and review, of all the good quality research studies on the use of garlic in people with high levels of cholesterol. The latest such meta-analysis was published in the *Annals of Internal Medicine* in 2000. As in the study just discussed, the results indicated a reduction in the levels of cholesterol of at least 10 percent, when small doses of garlic supplements were taken.

How Garlic Works against Cholesterol

According to scientists, such as David Kritchevsky at the world-famous Wistar Institute in Philadelphia, garlic specifically slows down the whole "production line" that makes the cholesterol in the liver. In addition, studies conducted by the U.S. Department of Agriculture show that garlic helps the liver to remove the excess cholesterol in the form of bile, and then eliminate the bile from the body. This is also the way certain mild, modern, cholesterol-lowering drugs work.

Garlic works immediately. In a study performed

smoking Seventh-Day Adventists, carried out in Holland in 1983, compared those who were vegetarians with those who were not, and found that the meat-eaters were three times more likely to incur a heart attack than the vegetarians. Vegetarians have more fiber in their diet. This, too, helps the arteries: As fiber passes through the digestive system, it absorbs fat and bile, and removes them from the body. In fact, the liver's function of making bile is one way the body eliminates excess cholesterol.

Hundreds of studies have demonstrated that animal fats have the unfortunate effect of increasing LDL cholesterol. Start to pay attention to the quantity and type of fats in your foods. Saturated fats, or hard fats, including animal fats, margarines, butter, and palm oil, all contribute to atherosclerosis and should be reduced. Switch instead to the many unsaturated vegetable oils now readily available in supermarkets, such as canola, soy, sunflower seed, or safflower oil. Your best choices for the heart are the monounsaturated oils, in particular olive oil. The use of olive oil, almost exclusively, in the Mediterranean diet is one of the reasons that the level of heart disease is so low in that part of the world. Be aware that even the highly unsaturated vegetable oils should not be used in excess, as they can reduce the levels of the "good" HDL cholesterol.

In Japan, which has the lowest heart disease level of all developed countries, dietary fat makes up around 12 percent of the total food intake; in the United States, where the heart disease rate is much higher, the percentage is three times as high.

Fat Is Just Part of the Problem

Fat is not the only dietary culprit in high cholesterol. Other dietary constituents, particularly sugar and alcohol, are converted into fat by the body.

Years of excessive alcohol or sugar consumption can keep the liver producing excess fat and sending it out into the circulation, adding to the LDL cholesterol.

Not everyone can switch from being a lifelong carnivore to a vegetarian overnight. But you can include more vegetables—preferably fresh ones—in your diet. Fresh leafy vegetables, fruit, nuts, and seeds are positive additions. All food fiber is helpful, especially the soluble fiber of fruit and vegetables. Food fiber ties up the excess cholesterol, ensuring that it is passed out of the body through the intestines. Fish and fish oil are also kind to the circulation. They thin the blood, helping to reduce cholesterol and also to discourage the clotting process.

Bile
A thick fluid secreted by the liver and stored in the gallbladder. It facilitates digestion of fats and helps to remove fats and cholesterol from the body as waste.

In addition, wholesome unprocessed foods are always healthier than refined and processed foods. For example, whole grains are better for our circulation than refined, white, bleached flour. Many essential micronutrients can be found eas - ily and inexpensively in natural, unrefined foods. When we choose whole grains, vegetables, fruit, nuts, and seeds, we add the antioxidants, such as vitamins C and E, as well as essential fatty acids, beta-carotene, zinc, copper, selenium, and magnesium into our diet.

Spices and herbs are a wonderful addition to your diet; they contribute health benefits and good taste to your foods. After all, it is among them that we find garlic.

The Stress Factor

Lifestyle is almost as important as diet. Moderate exercise, stopping smoking, and maintaining a normal weight all contribute to a healthy heart.

Stress is a major factor in causing raised blood cholesterol; if the body is under continuous stress, the liver makes extra cholesterol. It is dangerous to underestimate the threat to your health that stress creates. Researchers have found that people who were anxious, isolated, ambitious, or under a strain had a much higher chance of incurring heart attacks, even if they did not indulge themselves in doughnuts and hamburgers. This psychological dimension, along with other factors such as food quality and physical exercise, is seen as a reason why our ancestors were not bedeviled by heart disease, despite a fat-laden diet.

Garlic Is a Lifetime Health Aid

We've said that garlic starts working immediately. However, to receive more significant cholesterol-lowering benefits, you should continue to consume garlic for at least three months. You can continue taking garlic at the appropriate dosage for as long as the cholesterol problem persists; however, it would be best to make regular garlic consumption a permanent part of your diet, because once you stop taking garlic, the level of fat in the blood gradually returns to what it was before. Make garlic one of your life habits if you want to keep your cholesterol low and heart disease at bay.

How much garlic should you take? You should take a minimum of one clove per day. Studies show that the more garlic you take, the greater the benefit, so two or even three cloves a day would be preferable to one clove, especially if the cholesterol problem is severe. However, there is no need to take huge doses of garlic all at once, In fact, it is advisable to split the dose, taking half in the morning and half in the evening.

CHAPTER 3

GARLIC AND A HEALTHY HEART

Today a great deal more is known about garlic and its potential for improving our health. Our primary focus in this chapter is the fight against the leading cause of death in America—heart disease. We'll look at the various causes of heart disease and discuss in detail garlic's extraordinary power to lower blood pressure and thin the blood. In addition, we'll review various ways that garlic can protect the heart, slow down the process of heart disease, possibly even helping to reverse that process.

Heart Disease, a Major Health Problem

The good news is that we are living longer; the bad news is that diseases that build up over time will now reveal themselves. Heart disease, a cum - ulative condition, falls into the downside of the longer-life equation.

Consider the fact that 100 years ago, 75 percent of the people of Europe would not have reached their seventieth birthdays. Today, only one-third fail to make it. The big killers used to be infectious diseases, such as tuberculosis, diph - theria, venereal disease, cholera, and blood poisoning. Through developments in public health and sanitation, these diseases were subdued. But the victory over major diseases has only been partial.

Because people live longer, their risk of acquiring new kinds of diseases grows. Serious degenerative conditions of mid- and later life, like cancer and circulatory diseases, have replaced infectious diseases as the major threats to our health and well-being. Today, heart disease and cancer cause four out of every five deaths in middle age.

A Risk Factor Checklist

There is a gradual deterioration in our circulation over the years. This deteri-

Degenerative Diseases
Chronic health problems affecting us in later life, involving a reduction in normal function and resistance. Some examples are heart disease, cancer, and arthritis.

oration takes place because our modern lifestyle includes several factors that are known to affect the circulation. If any of these factors apply to you, you should consult a health professional to assess the condition of your heart and circulation and learn how to reduce the risk of damage that might occur in the future.

These risk factors are:

1. A high proportion of animal fats and other saturated or hydrogenated fats in the diet

2. Smoking

3. High blood pressure

4. High blood cholesterol

5. High blood sugar

6. Insufficient exercise

7. Obesity

8. Stress

There are secondary dietary factors to keep in mind as well. An imbalanced diet means a lack of crucial nutrients. You may not be getting enough of the proper vitamins and minerals, particularly the antioxidant vitamins such as C; E; magnesium; and B vitamins. A lack of these nutrients in your diet can contribute to heart disease.

How Our Circulation Becomes Clogged

Circulatory problems occur because our arteries collect streaks and lumps of fat on their inside surfaces, just as drains slowly become blocked by accumulating layers of waste.

The blockage to the arteries may start with slight damage to the artery lining. The damaged area attracts small cell pieces called platelets, which are a normal component of the blood that is involved in the clotting process. Once the platelets are attached, then sticky cholesterol globules, always present in the bloodstream, join the platelets. More and more cholesterol accumulates at the site and the result is a fatty deposit or plaque. In time, the deposits so swell the interior surfaces of the blood vessels that the passageway becomes partially blocked. The blockage is called a sclerosis, and the process of blockage is known as atherosclerosis.

When the sclerosis is severe, the fatty deposits precipitate the blood-clotting mechanism, normally reserved for sealing up cuts. Clots (known as thromboses) form inside the blood vessels. The vessels that seem to be most at risk are those that bring blood to the hardest-working muscle in the whole body—the heart. A clot that stops up these vessels prevents blood from reaching the heart, causing chest pain, angina, or if more severe, a heart attack.

Other blood vessels that are particularly vulnerable are those in the brain. If a thrombosis occurs here, it can lead to a stroke. Heart attacks and stroke are the most common effects of atherosclerosis. However, there can be other effects, such as an increase in blood pressure.

Proving That Garlic Works

The recent interest in garlic and the heart apparently came from doctors on vacation in the sunny Mediterranean. They were surprised to find that the population of the Mediterranean countries consumed large quantities of meat, smoked many cigarettes, and guiltlessly enjoyed their coffee in cafés all day long. Contrary to the doctors' expectations, these people did not have an exceptionally high incidence of heart disease. In fact, they were among the other countries, such as Japan, that have the lowest incidence of heart disease in the world.

A thorough and careful analysis by researchers at the University of Western Ontario in Canada found that the more garlic a nation consumed, the less heart disease there was among its population. And garlic is a major ingredient in Mediterranean cuisine.

However, scientists were reluctant to give all the credit for this phenomenon to garlic. After all, it was possible that other factors, such as the predominance of olive oil, fresh vegetables, and fruits in their diet played a role. Unrefined country food, as well as a more easy-going lifestyle, could be contributing to the low incidence of heart disease in Mediterranean countries. When asked, the people themselves insisted that garlic was responsible for their good health, but the scientists weren't so sure. They felt they needed more conclusive statistics.

The proof emerged in the form of a study conducted in India. Dr. Sainani and his colleagues at the Sassoon General Hospital in Pune, India, found the perfect subjects to test garlic, the Jains, members of a religious vegetarian Indian community. They all have a similar diet except that some are accustomed to eating onion and garlic, while others traditionally abstain from these foods. Dr. Sainani assembled three groups. One group consumed at least 21 ounces of onion and 1.75 ounces of garlic (this comes to around seventeen cloves—a fairly substantial quantity) weekly. The second group ate a weekly average of 7 ounces of onion and one-third ounce of garlic, and the third group ate no garlic or onion at all. It turned out that the amounts of cholesterol and fat in the blood of these individuals very closely matched the garlic and onion consumption. The heavy garlic eaters had 25 percent less cholesterol than the garlic avoiders. This decrease in cholesterol corresponds to a roughly 50 percent decrease in heart attack risk.

Garlic and Caring for Our Heart

Garlic can certainly help reduce the symptoms of heart disease. For example, Russian doctors have been using garlic preparations as a standard treatment for atherosclerosis, especially in the elderly. These doctors have reported improvement in symptoms, such as poor circulation in the legs and hands and tiredness, in many of their patients.

One relatively common and distressing problem that accompanies atherosclerosis is difficulty in walking due to an insufficient blood supply in the limbs (intermittent claudication). Garlic has been found to be very helpful in such cases. It enhances the effect of exercise, diet, and other treatments, although it works best before the problem has become very advanced.

A Note of Caution: Garlic will be most effective before your problem has become too severe. The sooner you start taking it, the easier it will be to prevent heart disease, or to remedy another already-existing problem. And it is important to repeat, garlic works best in conjunction with other means, such as medication or remedies prescribed by your health professional. Even once your symptoms have begun to resolve, it is important to keep taking garlic to prevent their return.

Garlic Can Help Lower Blood Pressure

When your heart pumps blood through your arteries, it creates pressure in the circulatory system.

Hypertension (high blood pressure) occurs when blood pressure stays elevated over time. An estimated 50 million Americans, about one in four adults, are suffering from high blood pressure.

High blood pressure can be a result of any number of factors, including excessive salt intake, excess bodily fluid, hormone imbalance, excessive coffee consumption, the presence of toxins in the body, lack of exercise, poor flexibility of the vessels, atherosclerosis, and stress. In some cases it is more difficult to reverse, and may require medication.

Whatever the cause, high blood pressure, or hypertension, increases the risk of heart problems, and should be taken very seriously. It may lead to congestive heart failure, heart attack, kidney failure, or stroke. Because high blood pressure produces few overt symptoms, doctors often call it the "silent killer." Normal blood pressure is around 120 when the heart contracts, and 80 when the heart relaxes. A blood pressure level of 140/90 millimeters of mercury or higher is considered high. About two-thirds of people over age sixty-five have high blood pressure.

Garlic's role here is to assist other remedies. It can reduce the blood pressure on its own by regular administration, to a limited extent, but not in everyone. Its effects are greater the higher the blood pressure is to begin with. People who have normal blood pressure are not affected. Generally, garlic should be combined with heart-saving self-care measures. If you think your blood pressure may be high, seek proper professional advice to find out why, so that you can determine the proper methods to use to correct it.

Researching Garlic and Blood Pressure

In one typical study, reported in the journal *Drug Research*, researchers gave twenty patients tablets equivalent to about half a clove of garlic a day.

These patients were compared to a similar group of patients who received a standard drug. Within two weeks, the two measures of blood pressure in the garlic group dropped from 176 to 164, and 99 to 85, a decrease of about 10 percent overall. The effect of the drug, on the other hand, was more or less the same. Symptoms such as headache, dizziness, buzzing in the ear, and insomnia were improved.

Fresh garlic, garlic oil, or other equally potent garlic products all are effective in reducing blood pressure. This was the conclusion of a team of British researchers who critically examined many published studies on blood pressure. Their report, published in the prestigious *Journal of The Royal College of Physicians* in 1994, gives the thumbs-up for garlic—it consistently reduced high blood pressure in all the studies; the higher the blood pressure was to begin with, the more it was reduced.

There is some uncertainty about how garlic acts on blood pressure. Up until the last ten years, it was thought that it cleaned up toxic substances that raise blood pressure. Today, however, evidence indicates that garlic affects the prostaglandins—hormone-like substances present in the blood vessels—that are in charge of opening, relaxing, or tightening them. If the ves - sels in the periphery of the body are relaxed, then there is less resistance to the blood flow. There is evidence that garlic does indeed increase the flow of blood in these smaller vessels.

Blood Pressure
The force of blood as it is pumped through the arteries; recorded as two numbers—the first, systolic pressure (as the heart beats) over the second, diastolic pressure (as the heart relaxes between beats).

What is particularly significant is that, unlike conventional medication, garlic reduces both blood pressure and blood fat. Modern drugs used to treat blood pressure are rather specific and do not

Thin Blood Benefits Everyone

There is no need to worry that garlic will reduce clotting too much. The clotting tendency of people in developed countries is already so high, due to our sedentary lifestyles and high fatty deposits in the blood, that most us can benefit from thinner blood. Garlic simply brings the clotting to a more normal level. Moreover, there is no evidence that people who eat a large amount of garlic in their daily diet have a problem with too much bleeding.

Nevertheless, it is important to note that if garlic is being taken along with aspirin and anti-coagulant drugs, the anticlotting effects can be magnified. This is not normally harmful, but in situations where clotting is essential, such as during surgery, taking garlic should be avoided.

Reversing Heart Disease

Most doctors have erroneously assumed that once arteries are blocked, they can never become unblocked. They believed that the only effective treatments for angina (chest pains), high blood pressure, and blocked arteries are drugs or surgery. Now, because of the publication of a landmark study by Dean Ornish, M.D., in the *Journal of the American Medical Association*, the medical world is starting to acknowledge that heart disease can be successfully treated without drugs or surgery. Dr. Ornish showed that blocked arteries can be gradually opened by a broad health program, including supplements such as garlic, mild fasts, relaxation, radical reduction of fats, a vegetarian diet, and aerobic exercise. Dr. Ornish also recommends group therapy to help deal with stress and the anxiety it creates. Nonetheless, a health problem that has been accumulating invisibly for many

Stress
A chronic state of tension and over-arousal. Signs of stress generally include anxiety, an inability to relax, burn out, addictions, and insomnia.

years, in some cases since youth, will not disappear overnight. A good start on the road to health should include garlic along with the lifestyle methods pioneered by Dr. Ornish.

Garlic as Part of a Prevention Plan

To some extent, garlic will help to prevent heart disease on its own, especially if it is taken over an extended period. However, it is unlikely that garlic alone will bring the risk of heart disease as low as it is for vegetarians or the people in Japan who follow a traditional diet. Garlic must be combined with lifestyle change to be really effective. For example, garlic will add to the cholesterol-lowering effects of a heart-healthy diet.

Professor E. Ernst of the University of Munich, published convincing results in the *British Medical Journal* from a study on groups of patients who had high levels of cholesterol (more than 260 milligrams/100 milliliters). One-half of the patients were given a low-calorie diet for four weeks, and had 10 percent less cholesterol at the end of the period. The other half took garlic supplements as well and achieved a further 10 percent reduction, enough to bring their cholesterol levels down to nearly normal levels.

We do not need to regard high blood pressure and heart attacks as more or less inevitable. After all, the Japanese do not suffer from atherosclerosis unless they immigrate to a Western country or consume a Western diet. People on these diets eat less than one-third of the fat that Westerners eat, and the traditional Japanese diet has no dairy products, meat products, sugar, bread, or cakes. The blood pressure of primitive people living in the wild goes down with age, not up. From very extensive reviews of who is, and who is not, vulnerable to heart disease several facts are clear. We can protect our hearts when we don't smoke; learn to live with less anxiety; exercise; eat a healthy balanced diet low in fat and containing plenty of fresh fruit and vegetables; and consume natural nutritious unprocessed foods. Such a lifestyle can make a tremendous difference in the way we feel too. Be sure to add some fresh garlic into your low-fat recipes to give your heart an extra boost.

CHAPTER 4

GARLIC—
THE DETOX HERB

In this chapter we'll look at the properties in garlic that, combined with the body's natural mechanisms, work to keep the body clean and poison free. We'll also review the many studies that point to garlic sulfur compounds as a protector against cancer—after heart disease, the nation's second biggest killer.

Problems of Toxins in the Body

Nearly every summer, in cities all over the industrialized world, there are days when we are warned not to leave our homes. We are cautioned that breathing the air is hazardous to our health. But no matter what the season, the pollution outside our walls is just the tip of the iceberg. If you take a moment and read the list of ingredients contained in the food packages in your kitchen, you will immediately see that the processed foods that we consume are chock-full of chemicals, the long-term effects of which are often unknown. It seems as if every week, some specialist alerts the media to the potential harm to humans from pollution in our water, food, or air. We are living in a world contaminated by a large number and variety of chemicals that our bodies are simply not equipped to deal with.

> **Detox**
> Short for detoxification; a process using natural methods such as fasting, herbs, water treatments, and vitamin supplements to remove unwanted and harmful substances from the body.

In fact, many of the diseases that plague mod-

spread of cancer and to stimulate the immune system, further strengthening the body's defense against cancer. Garlic may be effective in preventing the development of abnormal cells and in slowing the progression of established cancer cells.

As recently as December 29, 2003, researchers at the prestigious Weizmann Institute in Israel released a statement that its scientists had found a way to harness allicin, garlic's powerhouse healer, and use it to kill cancer cells in mice. Here's an excerpt from this exciting press release:

Weizmann Institute scientists have destroyed malignant tumors in mice using a chemical that occurs naturally in garlic. The key to the scientists' success lies in the development of a unique, two-step system for delivering the cancer-wrecking chemical straight to the tumor cells. Allicin, as the chemical is called, is the substance that gives garlic its distinctive aroma and flavor.

Science Links Garlic with Cancer Prevention

After decades of research and experiments, science is producing evidence suggesting that garlic is effective in the prevention of cancer and that garlic and related foods may play an important dietary role in inhibiting cancer growth.

Even in 1953, Dr. A. S. Weissberger of Case Western University in Cleveland, Ohio, suggested that the sulfur in allicin might protect against cancer by helping to remove cancer cells. He injected cancer cells into mice, some with and some without a small amount of allicin from garlic. The mice that were injected with the cancer alone lived for only sixteen days. The mice that were injected with a combination of cancer and allicin lived for six months. This study awakened some interest in the possibility of garlic as a preventive against cancer.

Professor Sydney Belman of the New York Medical Center found that he could prevent much of the expected growths in mice injected with cancer cells by giving mice diallyl sulfide, one of the group of sulfides that make up garlic oil.

Evidence from animal studies has sufficed to interest the National Cancer Institute in Bethesda, Maryland in garlic. The institute began a $20-million "designer foods" research program to see if adding components found in specific foods to the diet would help reduce the risk of cancer. Garlic was one of the food items selected for research, along with rosemary, licorice, and several others.

Although there is no direct evidence that garlic acts as a cancer preventive in people, there is indirect evidence. An intriguing study comes from China. Dr. Xing Mei of Shandong Medical College observed that the people of Guanshan County had stomach cancer rates of 3.5 per 100,000 people. In the neighboring Qixia County, the stomach cancer rates were more than ten times higher, at 40 per 100,000 people. After looking at their diet and lifestyle, the only difference he could find was that the people of Guangshan each ate, on average, about six cloves of garlic a day; those from Qixia ate none.

Another example is the Iowa Women's Health Study, an American study published in 1994 by Dr. K. Steinmetz and colleagues. The intake of 127 separate foods was monitored in 41,387 women. The doctors explored the diet of these women, as well as cancer cases that appeared among them. Of all the foods eaten, only garlic was clearly connected with a reduced risk of cancer. The women who consumed one or more servings of garlic per week were, on average, 50 percent less likely to develop colon cancer. A review of many such studies, published recently in the *American Journal of*

Clinical Nutrition, concluded that there was convincing evidence that garlic reduced the risk of cancers of the stomach and colon.

The general view today is that regular consumption of fresh fruits and vegetables can help prevent cancer, and that garlic is one of the most important components of a cancer-preventive diet. Studies involving cells, animals, and tissues, show clearly that fresh garlic, garlic oil, allicin, the sulfides, and most garlic compounds are effective.

How Garlic Works as a Cancer Preventive

It is not known specifically how garlic protects but it may involve blocking formation of cancer-causing compounds, stopping their ability to form tumors, or even inhibiting the growth of tumor cells. This follows work conducted by Professor Michael Wargovich at the University of Texas, whose group studied the effects of two major purified components of garlic—diallyl sulfide, which is soluble in oil, and S-allyl cysteine, which is soluble in water. He tested these compounds on animals with cancer and found that the tumors could be reduced by between 50 and 75 percent. These compounds were also able to completely protect other animals from the disease even when he deliberately tried to induce a particularly virulent form of esophageal cancer.

His work has received a lot of media attention. He found that garlic sulfur-containing compounds helped the liver to break down cancer-causing chemicals, and also may prevent cells from switching to cancer growth patterns. With this purer inner environment and a boost to the immune system, the body is better able to ward off cancer.

Garlic and Cancer Treatment

However, it should be stressed that until the topic of cancer treatment by garlic constituents is properly investigated, we would be wise to look at garlic, not as a cure, but as one of many ways we can protect ourselves from cancer.

For garlic to be an effective "treatment" of cancer, it must reduce and ultimately eliminate tumors, and there is not yet evidence that garlic can accomplish such a formidable task. The present consensus among scientists and herbalists is that garlic is not strong enough to be a sole treatment for cancer. There are other herbs, such as some Chinese herbs, which have stronger effects on the immune system. But as a preventive, garlic is well worth considering.

CHAPTER 5

GARLIC—
THE NATURAL
ANTIBIOTIC

G arlic was prized for its ability to prevent and treat infections long before the seventeenth-century Dutch lens maker, Anthony Leeuwenhoek, invented a microscope powerful enough to see tiny bacteria microbes. In the Middle Ages, French priests used garlic to protect themselves against the deadly bubonic plague, now known to have been caused by bacteria. During both world wars, European soldiers in the battlefield put crushed garlic directly on their wounds and ingested it to kill stomach infections. Knowing garlic's power to heal and strengthen, the workers who built King Tutankhamen's tomb staged what was the first recorded labor strike when their daily ration of garlic was withheld. Throughout history, nearly every culture, from ancient Chinese to colonial American, has used garlic for general health,.

Today, garlic is one of the best-selling preventive medicines in Europe, where it is accepted as safe and effective by both medical authorities and government officials. In fact, in Eastern Europe it is known as "The Russian Penicillin," because garlic products used to be the number-one remedy in Russia for use against all kinds of infections.

Now that we have reached a midway point in our guide it's time to turn our attention to the age-old use of garlic against the common infections of man. We'll examine how we can use this time-tested wisdom in our lives today. Before the arrival of modern antibiotics, infections were life threatening. Garlic was often used as a natural antibiotic and must have saved many lives at a time when even a cut finger could be lethal.

In this chapter we'll outline when and how to use garlic against these common infections. We'll also show you why, quite often, it is safer to use this alternative than to use conventional antibiotics.

Natural and Safe, Garlic Attacks Infections

Garlic fights infection by operating on two levels simultaneously. First, it kills the bacteria directly. Second, as is now known, garlic also stimulates the proper functioning of the immune system. Studies have shown that garlic stimulates the cells of the immune system to search for and fight invading bacteria. Certain types of infection-fighting white blood cells, called natural-killer cells, become more active after exposure to garlic.

Garlic's main use is in fighting infections that are not acute or immediately life threatening. It deals best with chronic and less dangerous infections such as sore throats, bronchitis, catarrh, sinusitis, gum infections, coughs, diarrhea, indigestion, mild gastroenteritis, cystitis, skin infections, boils, and so on. In these cases, the only solution offered by conventional, modern medicine—antibiotics—may not be worth the cost in side effects it incurs. Moreover, often these infections tend to recur, requiring repeated doses of antibiotics, which, over time, may make the side effects more serious and even encourage recurrence of the infection. Garlic is a milder, safer, and no less effective substitute.

Treating Sore Throats, Blocked Ears, and Chest Infections

Garlic is known worldwide as a remedy for chest complaints, especially troublesome and persistent coughs and bronchitis. Some years ago a Polish group at the Pediatric Institute of the Academy of

Medicine in Poznam, under the direction of Dr. T. Ratinsky, studied the effectiveness of garlic treatments on 382 children, whose ages ranged between three months and fifteen years. They obtained their best results with cases of recurrent catarrh (an inflammation of mucous membranes in the nose and throat, producing mucus), and chronic bronchitis.

Antibiotics
Drugs, such as penicillin, that were first invented during World War II, and that target bacteria. Like garlic, many antibiotics work because their chemical structure contains sulfur.

Today, in Russia and Eastern Europe, garlic is often used by professional doctors for cases for which antibiotics would be prescribed in the West. In 1965, during an influenza epidemic, the *Moscow Evening News* told everyone, "eat more garlic" and the government flew in a 500-metric ton emergency supply.

Backed by Science, Garlic Fights Infection

The extent of scientific research proving garlic's anti-infective power is greater than most people realize. The first person to demonstrate the enormous potency of garlic was the renowned Louis Pasteur in 1858. He grew a covering of bacteria in a laboratory culture dish, and then dropped garlic juice into the dish. The garlic juice killed all the bacteria around it. This type of experiment has been repeated continually over the years on both bacteria and yeasts, and hundreds of studies have been published. At the University of Londrina in Brazil, a 1982 study showed that garlic juice was highly effective against twenty-one kinds of bacteria that cause stomach problems, including *Salmonella*, *Proteus*, *Shigella* (the organism which causes dysentery), and colon bacteria. Garlic juice stopped the growth of the bacteria as effectively as antibiotics, such as penicillin.

A study at the University of California at Davis showed that a 1–20 dilution of dried garlic in water could kill *Salmonella* speedily. After only one hour, only 10 percent of the bacteria survived, and after just another hour, only 1 percent remained. The scientists looked for examples of bacteria that had become resistant to garlic, as usually happens with conventional antibiotic treatment. They were unable to find any.

Salmonella infections in food affect millions of people annually. Garlic is an obvious recourse. Included in the diet, garlic can help prevent any *Salmonella* present in food from causing a stomach infection in the first place. There are other studies, such as one published by Dr. Rees and colleagues in the *World Journal of Microbiology and Biotechnology*, that show that garlic selectively kills the bacteria that invade the digestive system, rather than the natural bacteria that live there normally.

Laboratory studies have shown that a very wide range of bacteria is sensitive to garlic and that the range is wider than that of commonly used antibiotics. The bacteria that cause throat, mouth, stomach, skin, lung, and other infections are particularly sensitive, as are those that cause food poisoning. Garlic also kills bacteria that have become resistant to other antibiotics.

Although there are hundreds of fascinating medical reports and studies on the success of garlic, even against such intractable infections as tuberculosis, they date from the pre-antibiotic era. Many of them are from Eastern Europe and Russia. Since the success of antibiotics, there have not been any modern clinical research studies of the use of garlic to treat bacterial diseases in humans.

Treating Fungus

Let's start with fungal and yeast infections. Usually these infections are treated by various antifungal drugs that take some time to work. These drugs can create even more side effects than antibiotics. The prescribed drugs used against ringworm and other prolonged fungal skin infections can inhibit the white blood cells, and in many cases work more slowly than an active treatment with garlic.

Fungal infections tend to be nagging and continuous rather than fast and dangerous, and so are very suitable for garlic's more gentle, persistent action. As we shall see, there is evidence that garlic may be just as strong as the usual antifungal drugs, and very wide in its field of action.

The fungal and yeast problems suitable for treatment by garlic include ringworm, athlete's foot, cystitis, thrush, vaginitis, and Candida infections. All are particularly irritating and hard to eliminate with modern medical treatments. Candida, in particular, is a very widespread and ever-increasing health problem. Like other fungal infections, it tends to recur because the previous use of antibiotics and steroids has harmed the body's immune system. A whole range of health problems may result from Candida infections, particularly in the intestines. These include allergies (Candida may damage the intestine, allowing allergy-causing materials to leak through), fatigue and debility, and blood sugar problems. Garlic is the ideal remedy, and is frequently prescribed by naturopathic doctors treating these problems.

When treating either fungal or bacterial infections, garlic should be used quite aggressively. The dose should be substantial. It is necessary to take several cloves a day for real anti-infective action. But, garlic should not be left to work alone against more persistent problems. Garlic should not be regarded as just another antibiotic, but used in a holistic way. Combining garlic with nutritional and other self-care measures does the job more effectively.

The basic anti-infective regimen involves fasting. Fasting need not entail a complete break with all foods. Just eating fruit and green salads for a few days will give a powerful boost to the immune system and help toward a cure. Along with fasting, it is useful to take drinks of hot lemon juice, preferably with 1 teaspoonful of grated fresh ginger and honey, or some hot cider vinegar with honey and some vitamin C. These drinks help to cleanse the body of toxins and speed transit of the immune components through the body. My own family uses this kind of regimen whenever we have an infection, and none of us has needed antibiotics for the last thirteen years.

Research Shows That Garlic Fights Fungus

There is also a great deal of scientific evidence concerning the wide range of garlic's anti-fungal effects. A classic study of the effect of garlic on Candida was carried out by Dr. Frank Barone and Dr. Michael Tansey of the University of Indiana in 1977. They showed that the amount of garlic extract needed to kill Candida was similar to the doses of modern antifungal drugs that are normally used.

Candida
A chronic yeast infection located in the blood and the digestive system, which causes a range of symptoms such as allergies, fatigue, and digestive disturbances.

There have been some initial studies on the use of garlic in the treatment of fungal infections, especially in animals, which were carried out in the 1980s. Candida infections were cured experimentally in chickens by adding garlic to their diet. The growth of ringworm and other skin fungal infections in rabbits was shown to be stopped imme - diately by putting garlic on the infection; these infections healed within fourteen days. (However, garlic had no effect on the infections when given to the rabbits in their food.) Garlic's ability to control all kinds of infections in livestock animals has long been noticed by farmers and animal breeders, and its veterinary use has quite a following today.

There is a certain amount of evidence for garlic's antifungal effects in humans, as well. For example, in a study at the Veterans Administration Medical Center in East Orange, New Jersey, the juice of 10 grams of garlic (three cloves) was given to volunteers. After a half hour, their blood serum was able to kill the Candida cells. In one surprising study, Dr. Neil Caporaso and colleagues at New Jersey Medical University fed large amounts of garlic to volunteers. After a while they took blood samples and found that the blood alone could kill fungi in a laboratory culture dish.

An interesting observation appeared in the *Medical Journal of Australia*. It was submitted by a doctor who had treated a member of his own family for ringworm on the arms. In the interests of science, he treated one arm with garlic and the other with an antifungal drug. The garlic-treated arm healed in ten days; the drug-treated arm took twice as long to heal.

Clearly, the active ingredient of garlic that principally achieves these antibacterial and antifungal effects is allicin, which is present in fresh garlic. Garlic oil has proved not to be as strong when tested in the laboratory.

Fighting against Viruses and Worms

There are no known drugs available for combating common viral infections. In these cases, a doctor will generally recommend making yourself more comfortable through home care. How often have we heard the advice, drink lots of liquids, take two Tylenol, and go to bed? For more serious viral infections, like shingles, there are drugs that are not only merely partially effective but also toxic.

On the other hand, growing evidence indicates

that garlic is effective against colds and viruses, not only bacterial infections. Especially encouraging, for example, was a small study of AIDS patients, in which the white blood cells were shown to be better able to cope with viruses after three months of regular garlic supplements. The question is how? Does garlic work on the infection itself, on the poisons that it produces, or on bolstering the body's immune defenses? Maybe it works because, as traditional medicine would say, it is fiery and induces sweating, which cleanses, cools, and helps the healing process. As in treatment for other conditions, garlic is more effective in combination with other antiviral treatments than it is by itself.

The use of garlic against worms and parasites also has a long history and has been mentioned in the very earliest of medical records. As with bacteria and yeasts, the reactive sulfur compounds attack the organisms invading the body, but are not dangerous to body tissue.

Garlic is recommended to combat pinworms or threadworms, and should be taken both orally and as a suppository. After someone has eaten garlic or used it as a suppository, large numbers of worms may be excreted. Parasites that live higher up in the digestive system are also affected by it, but a long-term persistent treatment with garlic may be necessary in order to dislodge them.

Recently garlic has been shown to be effective in killing the organism that produces amoebic dysentery. Although to date modern drugs are still the best treatment for this condition, Professor David Mirelman, of the Department of Parasitology at the Weizmann Institute of Science in Israel, believes that garlic could one day benefit the millions of amoebic dysentery sufferers around the world. Fresh garlic extract, or allicin by itself (but not garlic oil) is a powerful amoeba killer that is about one-tenth as potent dose for dose as the leading anti-amoeba drug. Not only does it have fewer side effects than regular, modern drugs, but it is cheap and can be grown in most areas.

When Not to Use Garlic

Garlic is appropriate for several different kinds of infections that are mild and not dangerous. However, if the infections become acute or grow serious, with signs like high fever and spreading inflammation, seek medical treatment. Do not ex -pect garlic to cure it.

More serious infections must be combated quickly and powerfully with modern drugs, such as antibiotics. Throughout history, because nothing else was available, garlic was used for serious infections such as tuberculosis, but today we have modern drugs that work very quickly and effectively to provide a cure.

Our Natural Pharmacy

Garlic has been shown to be weaker than antibiotics. If a specific amount of garlic juice is placed in the middle of a dish of bacteria, and its effect compared to that of a similar amount of a modern antibiotic such as penicillin, tetracycline, or erythromycin, garlic will be on average around one-tenth as strong. This is why it takes longer to work, and is only suitable for milder infections. But, al -though garlic may be slower, it does have a much wider range of action and can deal with almost any kind of bacteria. Antibiotics, on the other hand, are more specific and sometimes several drugs will have to be tried before the right one is found to kill a specific bacteria.

Garlic is like a shotgun, a wide range weapon. Antibiotics are like high-powered rifles designed to pinpoint specific targets. The main advantage in using garlic against infection is that it has no harmful side effects and the body never builds up a resistance to its healing powers. No matter how much or for how long you take garlic, it will never lose its ability to heal.

Though we do not need to turn the clock back and rely on garlic exclusively, it should still take pride of place in our kitchen's natural pharmacy.

CHAPTER 6

THE ESSENCE OF GARLIC

Garlic is a close relative of the onion and belongs to the lily family. Its botanical name is *Allium sativum* and is part of the allium group of plants in which there are some 600 species. Many of garlic's relatives are familiar to us. Onion, chives, leeks, and shallots are just a few of the species we use regularly in cooking. Garlic, whose name comes from the Anglo-Saxon word *garleac*, meaning spear-leek, has a solid, round, smooth stem and narrow, flat spearlike leaves. Clusters of purple-white flowers grow from the stems, which can be as high as two feet.

The graceful leaves originate from the fleshy, fat base of the stem, which is the head (or bulb) of garlic that grows below ground. This bulb, when dried, is the garlic you find in the supermarket. It usually contains eight to fourteen cloves, each one enclosed in a thin, white, papery covering. These small cloves contain the powerful ingredients that can improve our health.

Garlic is grown from its own clove (see Chapter 8 for growing instructions), and a great deal of it is grown and consumed worldwide. According to a United Nations' trade statistic, enough garlic is grown to give each member of the human race half a clove a day. China is the biggest producer, followed by India, Spain, and various Mediterranean countries. Here in the United States, garlic growth has soared, hitting a record-high of 3.1 pounds per person in 1999. No other vegetable has had stronger growth demand over the past ten years. That's quite a lot of garlic for a country that views garlic as the most distasteful smell among foods. Ninety percent of American's garlic is grown at home, much of it in Gilroy, California, the "Garlic Capital of America." In the harvest season, you don't need a map to get to Gilroy, just follow your nose! The annual garlic celebration, a twenty-five-year-old tradition, has become a joyous gathering of garlic aficionados from all over the United States.

Weights and Measures

Like most vegetables, garlic is mostly water, 60 percent to be exact. A clove, which may only weigh about one-eighth of an ounce, contains approximately 1 gram of carbohydrates, 0.2 grams of protein, a little fat, and small amounts of B-complex vitamins, vitamins C and E, plus the antioxidant mineral selenium. This nutrient is an important part of the antioxidant enzymes that protect cells against the effects of free radicals, which are produced during normal oxygen metabolism. Garlic is the richest source of selenium among the edible plants, but because it is eaten in such small quantities, its selenium contribution to the diet is minimal. The other vitamins and nutrients obtained from garlic are similarly in-significant.

Garlic's Medicinal Ingredients

Garlic contains some remarkably strong and unique substances. These are the substances that can keep our arteries open and kill bacteria, yeasts, and fungi. These remarkable substances have one element in common: sulfur. However, it is the large amount of a particular and very unusual sulfur compound that is found in each garlic clove that is the key to garlic's healing power. That compound is called alliin.

Alliin constitutes from 0.3 to 1 percent of the

weight of garlic, although it makes up in power what it lacks in quantity. The amounts of alliin, and the consequent amount of the active sulfur compounds, can vary extensively in different garlic bulbs grown in different fields, in different countries, and under different culti-

Bulb

The fleshy base of the stem of the garlic and similar plants (like the lily, onion, or tulip) that is the underground storage of the nutrients needed for next year's growth.

vation methods. For example, Chinese garlic is quite rich in active ingredients, as is garlic that is grown organically (in soil that has not been chemically treated). Research suggests that certain bacteria in the soil are important in making sulfur compounds from the earth available to the hungry roots of the garlic plant.

The Discovery of Garlic's Power

Like all scientific discoveries, the main secrets of garlic's strength began as a puzzle. How is it that a clove of fresh garlic, when intact, has no smell or taste? Yet, the moment it is crushed or cut, the strong smell and familiar garlicky taste attack the senses.

The answer was found in 1944 by scientists working for the Winthrop Chemical Company in the United States. Researchers there found that the alliin in a garlic clove when crushed or chop-ped mixes inside the garlic tissues with a catalytic agent called allinase. The chemical reaction be-tween the two changes the alliin into yet another compound called allicin and produces the strong smell and fiery taste. Allicin is the substance that burns the tongue when you bite into a fresh clove of garlic. The burning sensation gives us an idea of what all those strange compounds are doing in the garlic bulb in the first place. Powerful allicin is the garlic plant's defensive chemical weapon against any marauding pest foolish enough to try and take a bite out of it!

Once Created, Allicin Begins to Heal

After crushing, garlic becomes a powerful, complex mix of substances. Allicin is highly reactive and it changes of its own accord into a range of other sulfur compounds, mainly sulfides. These sulfides give garlic its heavy smell. Sulfides form rapidly when garlic is heated as in cooking. If crushed garlic is left standing in or out of the refrigerator, sulfides form more slowly, in about an hour or so.

Sulfur
A natural element that is often found in pungent foods, such as onion, radish, and garlic, that can have a powerful therapeutic effect on the body.

After much debate over the years, it has now been conclusively proved that allicin is the main active medicinal compound in garlic. It has been known for over fifty years that if you take allicin out of garlic and use it in simple laboratory tests to kill bacteria and fungi, it will do so just as well as the whole crushed garlic. However, if garlic is boiled or treated so there is no allicin, it actually helps the growth of bacteria, rather than prevent it. This has been confirmed many times, and even the Nobel Prize winner in Chemistry, Artur Vitaanen, has shown that allicin must be present for garlic to work.

In studies at the Department of Microbiology at the University of Indiana, many garlic compounds were checked to see how they rated as natural antibiotics. Only allicin, or the sulfide daughter compounds created when allicin breaks down, were effective.

The same picture emerges in relation to the effect of garlic on the circulation and cholesterol levels. To date, virtually all of the thirty-five clinical studies carried out on garlic and the circulation used fresh, dried, or distilled garlic containing allicin and/or its sulfide daughter compounds. A team of researchers at the United States Department of Agriculture Laboratories in Madison, Wisconsin, have tested many different extracts of garlic for their ability to help lower cholesterol levels. All these studies were conclusive. Only those extracts that contained or had contained allicin were effective.

When Allicin Enters the Body

Scientists are now beginning to have some idea of what happens to garlic's powerful chemicals once they enter the body. When you eat crushed garlic or garlic powder, you are taking in a combination of allicin and its precursor substances including some remaining alliin that has not yet been converted to the active allicin compound.

In the intestine, this leftover alliin is probably all converted to allicin. Then the allicin begins to pass through the walls of the digestive tract into the body where it enters the bloodstream. The blood takes the allicin to the liver where it is processed into sulfides. It is converted in a similar way as when crushed garlic is cooked. The sulfides spread throughout the body, healing and purifying. Within a few hours, after they've done their work, the sulfur compounds formed from the allicin are excreted in the urine.

There's More: Additional Garlic Constituents

Like all natural herbal remedies, garlic contains a galaxy of chemical substances, most of which effect our bodies. True, allicin is the most important substance in garlic in terms of its medicinal power. But there are many others.

One interesting group, which includes a compound called ajoene, was researched by Professor Erick Block of the State University of New York at Albany, and reported in an article in the *Scientific American*. Ajoene and related compounds are created when garlic is fried or crushed in oil or when it is crushed and mixed with alcohol in the laboratory. Dr. Block's research found these mixtures to be very powerful anticlotting substances.

There are also small quantities of compounds based on the amino acid cysteine. Garlic is a close relative of the onion. Not only does garlic contain substances that taste and smell like onion, but onion creates substances similar to allicin, when it is cut or crushed—the substances that make you cry.

Garlic, with its sulfurous nature, is clearly both fierce and friendly. As we'll see later on in the guide, garlic is viewed in folk tradition as a little bit of hell that brings a little bit of heaven. Let's see how we can harness its hellish strengths and make the best use of its healing properties.

CHAPTER 7

GARLIC'S HISTORY AND GLOBAL HEALING

Like all our herbal remedies and medicinal foods, garlic is part of a precious human inheritance. With the growing interest in herbs and natural remedies, garlic is taking on a new and important place in the way we approach healing.

Although this guide deals primarily with today's important findings and clinical studies, the rich history of garlic as a food and health aid has also contributed much to our knowledge of it. In this chapter we'll take a look at the fascinating role garlic has played throughout history from the courts of kings to the hovels of the common people. Also, we'll discuss traditional uses of garlic for man's circulatory health and the present-day holistic physician's attitudes toward its role in various treatment programs.

From Ancient Egypt to Your Pharmacy Shelves

Tomb raiders may be looking for precious gold and scrolls, but one item they can count on finding is garlic! Dating from the time of the early pharaohs, more than 6,000-year-old Egyptian burial grounds at El Mahasana were rich with little clay models of garlic bulbs. Along with the abundant gold and jewels in the tomb of King Tutankhamen, six perfectly dried bulbs were found; perhaps they were there to give him sustenance during his long journey through the afterlife. The ancient Egyptians clearly appreciated garlic, both for its flavor and as an important medicine. Inscriptions on the

Great Pyramid give an account of the large amounts of garlic consumed by the laborers. In what must be one of the oldest medical texts, the Ebers Papyrus, there is a list of twenty-two garlic recipes for boils, stomach infections, infected glands, and overall body weakness.

The fare of ancient kings, garlic was also relied on for taste, strength, and nourishment by the common folk. The Jews in the wilderness, according to the Bible (Numbers 11:46), became so bored with their monotonous diet of manna that they longed for the garlicky food of Egypt, even though they had eaten it as slaves. Like their modern compatriots, the ancient Greeks loved their garlic, too. Aristotle, a mathematician and the Western world's most influential philosopher, recommended garlic as a tonic. Garlic is even blamed for starting the Trojan War, which led to the fall of Troy. According to the story, some young Greeks "primed with garlic" stole a princess, and so the war began and continued for many years. Powerful stuff, indeed.

Roman legions planted it wherever they were stationed, in vegetable plots beyond the walls of their camps. They believed that it made them fighting fit and more aggressive.

Follow the Ancient Doctors' Recommendations

Throughout history, garlic has been valued as a medicine as well as a food. Hippocrates, often called the father of modern medicine, praised garlic for driving out excess water from the body, settling upset stomachs, and curing infections and inflammations. Here is one of his remedies for an infected lung: "And if you recognize the signs of suppuration (pus), the sick man, for his evening meal and before he goes to bed, should eat raw garlic in great quantity and should drink a noble and pure wine. If by this means the pus erupts, so much the better."

Dioscorides, the Roman physician whose understanding of plants has been the inspiration of herbalists right up to the present day, had this to say about garlic: "Garlic makes the voice clear, and soothes continuous coughing when eaten raw or boiled. Boiled with oregano, it kills lice and bed bugs. It clears the arteries. Burnt and mixed with honey, it is an ointment for blood-shot eyes: it also helps baldness. Together with salt and oil, it heals eczema. Together with honey, it heals white spots, herpetic eruptions, liver spots, leprosy, and scurvy. Boiled with pinewood and incense, it soothes toothache when the solution is kept in the mouth. Garlic with fig leaves and cumin is a plaster against the biting of the shrew-mouse . . . A mush from crushed garlic and black olives is a diuretic. It is helpful in dropsy."

Other Greek and Roman authorities added to the list of the medical problems that might be successfully addressed through the use of garlic. This list includes tumors, and parasites such as those that cause malaria, and ear infections. Galen, one of the true fathers of medicine, called it "countryman's cure-all" and Gaius Pliny, the greatest natural historian of ancient times, compiled an astonishing list of up to fifty disorders that garlic could cure. Pliny died observing the eruption of Vesuvius, which buried Pompeii—in whose ashes garlic was, of course, found preserved.

Hippocrates

Known as the father of medicine, this Greek physician was actually the father of natural healing. Over 2,000 years ago his books recommended healthy eating, natural living, and remedies such as garlic.

In the Medieval World

Throughout medieval and Renaissance Europe, garlic was a familiar part of life, and its smell was a part of the fun. A contemporary source mentions how Henry IV of France, who ruled from 1589 to

1610, chewed garlic and had "a breath that would fell an ox at twenty paces." Imagine what he could do to his enemies at court! At the same time, garlic's health-giving qualities were praised by all the leading herbalists. According to their theory of elements and humors, garlic was regarded as very "heating and drying," and was therefore used to combat "moist" and "cold" diseases, including catarrh and boils, various stubborn infections, and sluggish circulation of the blood. According to William Turner, the herbalist of English queen Elizabeth I, it "maketh subtill the nourishment and the blood," implying that it has cleared blockages in both. This statement is of great interest to us today as we research garlic's role in combating high cholesterol and blood clots.

The Fall from Favor

By around 1600 a prejudice against garlic's pungency began to develop in northern, Protestant Europe. Garlic became one of the signs of class distinction; it was now regarded as the food of rustics and peasants, and not suited to the refined palates of the upper classes. In Shakespeare's *Measure for Measure*, act 2, scene 2, Lucio says of the Duke that he would "mouth with a beggar though she smell (of) brown bread and garlic."

In 1699, in his book on salads, the famous diarist John Evelyn wrote of garlic, "We absolutely forbid its entrance into our salleting [salad making] by reason of its intolerable rankness."

Spaniards, Italians, and French people might eat it, so might peasants—especially if they lived in damp places—and sailors, but garlic was definitely beneath the dignity of English ladies and gentlemen. During the nineteenth century, this trend was well expressed by the culinary and domestic guru of those days, Mrs. Beeton. As she wrote in her *Book of Household Management*, considered the cookbook/bible for Victorian respectability, "the smell of the plant is generally considered offensive . . . It was in greater repute with our ancestors than it is with ourselves, although it is still used as a seasoning or herb."

The growing prejudice against garlic spread with the Northern Europeans to the United States, where it is still widespread. Surveys conducted on the subject of tastes always seemed to find that garlic is the most unpopular flavor of all, along with olive oil. Now it may be hard to imagine, but at the top of the list were bananas, chocolate, and strawberries!

How did these prejudices come about? They arose because aristocratic people began to express their refinement through a new, starched cleanliness. Pungent smells became the province of the poor: for the rich it was all lavender and roses. As time went on, bland tastes and odors became associated with self-discipline, primness, and restraint. The Victorians in England rarely ate garlic. Perhaps those subscribing to the Puritan ethic in America also wanted to disassociate themselves from anything that might remind them of the passionate nature of the Mediterranean peoples or with the "repellent" grubbiness of the working classes.

Thankfully, a change is coming about. Today, the health-conscious middle and upper classes eat garlic, along with brown, whole-wheat bread, and other natural foods. The old, bland, inoffensive cooking is seen as inhibited and even uncultured, as well as irrelevant to the way we live today. Accompanying the return to a natural lifestyle is an acceptance and appreciation of the rich aromatics of herbs, spices and, of course, garlic.

Healing Folk Traditions

Among the common folk, garlic was seen as an energy-producing food and was regarded as a general tonic. Folk practitioners all over the world have always used it. For example, traditional midwives in the Middle East gave garlic to women for ten days after childbirth to prevent infections and build their strength.

Gypsies are famous users of garlic. One of their classic medicines for a cough is fresh garlic boiled in milk. Russian folk medicine suggests garlic and onion mixed with honey or vinegar as a general health tonic, especially for the elderly. There are also uses that strike us, with our modern sensitivities, as peculiar. Most folk traditions regard garlic as aphrodisiac, but today potential lovers might not agree because of the odor!

Use of Garlic for the Heart in Folk Medicine

In Asian—and especially Indian—medicine, garlic was specifically used to remove fat from the blood and to dry out excess moisture from the body. Indian medical sources noted that it reduced the amount of milk produced by breast-feeding mothers, and they advised them to be careful of their garlic consumption. Thousands of years ago, Charaka, the traditional father of Indian medicine, stated that garlic maintains the fluidity of the blood and strengthens the heart, and traditional Indian physicians nowadays rely on garlic and onion therapy to prevent heart disease.

Dioscorides, and William Turner after him, prescribed garlic against "blockages" or "stiffness" of the blood system. The relatively common disease known as "dropsy," in which part or all of the body swelled up and became "waterlogged," arose from poor circulation. Today, we know this condition as edema. Early English doctors talk of garlic's heat as "boiling away the fluid" of dropsy, and garlic became the principal treatment for this condition.

The old herbalists said that garlic worked be - cause of its heating and drying properties, which removed water from the body and opened "cold," atrophied, and blocked blood vessels. Today, of course, we would call the condition of these blocked vessels atherosclerosis, and speak of diseases of the circulation, which means much the same thing. Thus, there is an ancient precedent for garlic and its role in keeping our hearts healthy.

Garlic as a Folk Medicine against Infections

Early practitioners of herbal medicine recommended garlic for infections of the stomach, mouth, throat (such as sore throat, coughs, and catarrh), ears, and skin. It was used both internally and externally for boils, acne, carbuncles, and ulcers. As we mentioned before, during World War I it was used extensively by both sides to treat infected wounds. In the British trenches, sterilized sphagnum moss containing garlic juice was generally placed over an injury. Reports from that time describe it as a successful front-line protection against gangrene. It was also used in the trenches against dysentery, a practice continued during World War II in the countries of Eastern Europe.

Traditional Medicine
Refers to the rich, accumulated medical wisdom of various cul-tures throughout the world, often going back thousand of years.

Garlic has been used against some very ugly infections indeed. Very large doses, or "saturation doses," were used, with some effectiveness, to treat tuberculosis and leprosy. It was also used against cholera and typhoid with considerable success. Dr. Albert Schweitzer used garlic in this way in Africa. Even the plague, while not cured by garlic, may have been deterred by it. French garlic-loving priests who attended the bedsides of victims in eighteenth-century London remained healthy, while the non-garlic-eating English priests succumbed.

For those bitten or stung by the nastier little friends in the animal kingdom, garlic was used as a natural first-aid balm. Aristotle recommended it for rabies and Mohammed for scorpion stings. I can vouch for its usefulness in the case of a certain common, nonlethal, but still unpleasant Middle Eastern scorpion. Greek and Roman herbalists called it an antidote to snakebite, and told how farmers would carry it with them in the fields.

As for country cures, even today organic farmers and pet owners recommend garlic in caring for cows, sheep, and horses for many of the same illnesses that humans suffer from, including worms, and digestive and skin infections.

Magic and Mystery

Almost all of us have seen the old vampire movies where peasants kept braids of garlic in their humble huts to ward off a visit from their friendly neighborhood vampire. Throughout Eastern Europe, this kind of garlic legend abounds; even today, garlic is put on a woman's pillow during childbirth and in a child's clothes during baptism.

A possible explanation for the supposed role that garlic plays in magic and superstition probably corresponds to its invaluable use against common infections. At a time when no one knew that infections were caused by bacteria and viruses, it was assumed that diseases were passed on by evil spirits. Since garlic could prevent and cure diseases, maybe it could chase away the spirits that caused them.

There is another perhaps even more interesting reason for the superstitious beliefs behind garlic. One Islamic legend suggests that when Satan was thrown out of paradise, garlic grew on the ground first touched by his foot. This fanciful tale points to the apparent paradox of garlic. On the one hand, garlic contains almost heavenly properties. It purifies, cleanses, and detoxifies the body. It cures diseases and adds flavor to foods. On the other hand, there is something hellish about it too. The odor can be unpleasant and the flavor sharp and overwhelming.

The Herbalist's View

Today's health practitioners use garlic to address an array of physical problems, most of which have been covered in this guide. For example, it was herbalists that showed the scientists that garlic thins the blood. Holistic physicians in India, practicing the Indian system of medicine, have always administered garlic to people with too much fat in their bloodstream. In China, people use it a great deal for worms, parasites, and stomach infections. Asian medical doctors also prescribe garlic plasters for boils and garlic in combination with other herbs for all kinds of infections. Modern herbalists prescribe garlic products for almost all circulatory problems and fresh extracts of garlic for bronchial infections, tonsillitis, abscesses, Candida, and other infections.

CHAPTER 8

GARLIC IN YOUR KITCHEN AND GARDEN

A s I've discussed, garlic was shunned for centuries and because of its strong flavor and odor, was considered a low-class, peasant seasoning, only winning wide acceptance in cooking outside working-class kitchens after World War II. Today, you can step into the cooking section in any bookstore and you'll find dozens of cookbooks dedicated to garlic. From the simple combination of the Greek mainstay of *tzadziki* made with fresh garlic, yogurt, and chopped cucumbers, to elaborate dishes of roasted brisket with garlic, onions, and plums, you'll find that garlic is enjoying a renaissance in modern sophisticated cuisine.

Whether it is for health or flavor, there is a staggering range of dishes that can be improved by adding garlic. In this chapter we'll explain several different ways to take your garlic in tasty and healthy recipes. Then, we'll describe how to deal with the odor of garlic, and finally we'll give you overall advice on how to grow it in your garden.

Garlic Odor
Arises from its sulfur-containing compounds, which are also the medicinally active ones, and cannot be easily avoided in fresh garlic.

For Best Health Benefits, Keep Cool

Does garlic keep its medicinal potency in the cooking pot? In principle, garlic will still work if we cook it, providing we crush it first. This is necessary to release the active allicin compounds. However, the health benefits of garlic and other medicinal foods are partly destroyed by the high temperatures of cooking. Also, the longer the food is cooked, the smaller the quantity of medicinal ingredients that will be left at the end of the process. Those ingredients not destroyed by the heat will be released into the air and lost, filling the room with the rich, spicy aromas of healthy ingredients that should have been in the pot. Therefore, the way to derive the greatest benefit when cooking with garlic is to add it close to the end of the cooking process.

To guarantee that we get the full dosage and medicinal benefit from garlic and other spices, it may be necessary to take them separately from food. As a general rule, you can regard spices within food as having a mild preventive effect, and spices taken separately from food as having a stronger medicinal action. For example, a few seeds of fennel in your vegetable soup will have a gentle, calming effect on your digestion, but fennel tea will be more effective in treating stomach gas. Similarly, garlic used in cooking will have a mildly positive effect on your circulation, but if you have a cholesterol problem, you should take an appropriate dose of garlic either fresh or in supplement form.

Some Powerful Garlic Cooking Tips

Vegetarians can make use of garlic in hundreds of dishes. Garlic goes well with almost any soup, including vegetable broth. It can be crushed and added in mid-cooking to enrich the taste of pies and quiches as well as stews and casseroles. A combination of olive oil, garlic, and rosemary is one of the more delicious ways to add garlic to potatoes and other root vegetables. Garlic is wonderful in pickles, sauces, mushroom dishes, and salad dressings. A classic vinaigrette made with olive oil, lemon, cider vinegar, garlic, mustard, and herbs is a delicious addition to a bowl of fresh salad greens. Try a garlic, lemon soy-sauce dressing on fresh vitamin filled avocado for a delicate, healthy side dish.

Whole-grain breads, pastas, and crackers taste great with garlic-flavored spreads and sauces. A classic Middle Eastern dip that is superb for the circulation consists of a mix of olive oil, squeezed lemon, garlic, and marjoram. Use garlic in pasta sauces whether tomato or olive oil based. Enjoy freshly cooked pasta tossed lightly with virgin olive oil and finely chopped fresh garlic. Garnish with some fresh parsley and you'll enjoy a classic taste of Italy and all the health benefits of fresh garlic.

In Spain and in Italy, different versions of bruschetta are enjoyed by spreading fresh crushed garlic, olive oil, and some finely chopped tomatoes on fresh whole-grain bread before warming it in the oven. This is a healthier version of the old garlic butter.

Garlic is a welcome addition to lean meat, especially in French garlic-based sauces. Crushed garlic, parsley, and lemon make a deep and sophisticated sauce for broiled, grilled, and baked fish. A little garlic is a wonderful addition to bean and lentil dishes. Add crushed garlic and dill to curd and cream cheeses to give them a rich, aromatic flavor. Humus and tahini, the Middle Eastern dips that are served all over Europe and America these days, are made with chick peas and sesame seeds, and their main flavor ingredient is garlic.

In Indian and Chinese cooking, garlic is fried in oil, often with onion. The oil is then used as the basis for numerous dishes, such as curries and stir-fries.

When it comes to garlic and cooking you are only limited by your imagination.

Your Kitchen Drugstore: Fresh Garlic Remedies

For maximum medicinal effect, take fresh garlic. It

should be crushed and left standing for a couple of minutes to allow the allicin to form. Then add it to a quantity of warm water or milk, to fruit such as apples and pears, to vegetable juices or soups, or to green salads such as lettuce and parsley. All of these methods will help to eliminate the burning sensation in the mouth or stomach. There are hundreds of ways to prepare garlic. Here are some classics:

Garlic in Milk

Crush one clove in half a cup of warm milk. Add honey to taste. This is an old gypsy remedy. Since cow's milk is not the best drink to take during chest or throat infections, or where there is mucus, this remedy can be modified by using soy or rice milk.

Garlic Syrup

Pharma-copoeia
The official list and guide to drugs published by government health departments.

This is similar to the garlic syrups described in official drug guides, such as the British pharmacopoeia, in the early twentieth century. It is recommended by many herbalists. The garlic is not fresh, as in other recipes, but it seems to keep its power remarkably well.

Put 250 grams (about ten heads or eighty cloves) of crushed garlic in a 1 liter jar. Almost fill the jar with cider vinegar and water in equal amounts, cover and leave for a few days, shaking occasionally. Strain through a cloth, add 1 cup of honey, stir, and keep in the refrigerator. This syrup will keep for up to a year. It is especially useful for coughs, nasal and bronchial problems, and sore throats, as well as for circulatory problems. One tablespoon a day is the correct dose.

Garlic and Miso Soup

Miso, a Japanese soybean extract, makes an ex-cellent hot soup, ideal to take with garlic. Dissolve a teaspoonful of miso in just-boiled water. Add a couple of drops of soy sauce, a good squeeze of lemon, some grated onion, and one or two crushed cloves of garlic. This is especially good during the convalescent period of an infection, as it brings strength as well as healing. A concentrated vegetable stock can be substituted for the miso.

External Applications of Fresh Garlic

In some situations garlic needs to be applied directly to the skin or mucosal surfaces to be effective. Athlete's foot, fungal infections, stings, Candida in the urogenital area, and tooth and gum infections are conditions that respond to topical garlic treatment. Unless the skin is overly sensitive, one can simply crush garlic onto a small piece of cotton and bind it directly to the infected area. There may be some burning sensation, which passes in a few minutes. The garlic can be retained on the affected area by spreading Vaseoline or hand cream around the area. If the burning would otherwise be too intense, on the gums, for example, you can use a slice of garlic that has been left for thirty minutes after crushing because it weakens with exposure.

Garlic in Your Spice Rack

It is easy to add the rich taste of garlic to your food by just reaching for a container filled with one of the many varieties of processed garlic on your spice rack. Garlic can be powdered, granulated, minced, or combined with salt—all these forms add flavor, but they don't add much health benefit. They tend to be too processed and too old. However, frozen crushed garlic is readily available and very beneficial. The standard method of making frozen garlic is to crush the cloves and then freeze. When you use this kind of garlic, you'll be benefiting from the released allicin.

Dealing with Garlic's Odor

Now that you've had an introduction to garlic in cooking and learned how to take fresh garlic as a medicine, let's discuss the antidotes to the garlic breath that healthy self-care brings.

Most garlic breath comes from chewing garlic in the mouth, so the best way to avoid the problem is by eating it without chewing it. Fresh garlic can be crushed into milk as we described previously and thereby swallowed it one big gulp. Then there are foods that will neutralize the odor. Eating parsley or lettuce after your garlic consumption can remove much of the odor. You can also chew a few seeds of fennel or anise or drink mint tea. These breath remedies should be eaten or drunk with, and after, the garlic. You can find some creative ways to make garlic suit your habits.

One day, a visitor to my house was amazed to see my daughter, who was then six years old, cutting cloves of garlic into long slices. Then, with great concentration, she inserted them into grapes.

"What on earth are you doing?" he asked.

"Preparing my medicine," she answered, and popped one into her mouth.

These methods will prevent the odor of garlic from affecting the mouth, but there is still some odor that emerges from the skin and digestion. This cannot be avoided, but it is milder. The only way that this smell can be drastically reduced is by taking garlic products and supplements rather than fresh garlic. For many of us, this is a very convenient way of healing the heart and dealing with the nose at the same time.

Garlic in Your Garden

Garlic is a welcome addition to any home garden. It is very easy to grow in practically any climate, and needs very little care. Successful crops of garlic can be found from the cold of the Catskill

Mountains to the dry heat of New Mexico. In fact, the very properties that make garlic such a successful antibacterial agent for people can help neighboring plants in your garden stay healthy and grow more hearty. Here are some general tips on planting and harvesting your own crop of this healing medicinal plant.

When to Plant

Many garlic growers claim that it is best to plant garlic on the shortest day of the year and harvest on the longest. But any time in the late fall through to early winter is fine to plant your crop.

Soil Tips

No matter what the climate, you will need rich, fertile, and well-drained soil. Thoroughly decayed compost is beneficial, too. If you prefer, you can condition your soil a week or two before planting. If your soil tends to be acidic, add some lime to it. Add some sand, if your soil tends to be clayish.

Compost
Consists of collected and piled organic garden and kitchen waste matter, such as vegetable peels and leaves, which ferments naturally; the decaying process produces a fertilizer rich in natural nutrients.

Planting

Garlic is reproduced by breaking the head, or bulb, of garlic into individual cloves, which are then planted. Each clove you plant grows and eventually becomes a full new head of garlic. Choose the biggest and fattest seed cloves and sow them root end down, standing erect, about 2 inches (5 cm) or so under the soil surface. Place them about 4 inches (100 mm) apart. The distance between the rows should be 12 to 18 inches. Garlic plants thrive with a lot of sun. As a general rule, the plants should be well watered about once a week.

Harvesting

When most of its foliage has dried off, usually nine

months after planting, your garlic is ready to harvest. However, the state of the foliage is the indicator of readiness, not any particular date. Wash the bulbs, especially the roots, and leave them for a week or so to dry. When the bulbs are dry, you can trim off the roots, remove the outer peel, and hang up your garlic for storage.

Storage

Once you have harvested your garlic, tie it together by the stalk. Hang the garlic bundles in a cool dry place, out of the sun and where they can get adequate ventilation. Hang decorative braids of garlic in the kitchen. Or keep a small supply in one of the many attractive garlic jars now on the market.

Share the Goodness of Garlic with Companion Planting

Companion planting refers to growing different compatible plants together that are mutually beneficial. The main benefit of garlic is its natural-killer properties against fungus and garden pests.

Since there are over 300 strains and five varieties of garlic, it's best to check with your local nursery for specific growing instructions. But as you can see in our brief outline, garlic is simple to grow and a single season harvest can yield an invaluable crop.

Besides the obvious benefits of saving money and ensuring that your garlic is as fresh and natural as possible, the additional value of planting garlic in your garden is the reward to your spirits, of knowing that you are caring for yourself with your own natural medicines.

CHAPTER 9

GARLIC
SUPPLEMENTS

As we've seen, garlic is as effective a remedy as some modern drugs. However, garlic is a plant—a natural medicinal food. Because it is not a pill containing a precise amount of pure, regulated chemicals, garlic requires more attention from you.

In this chapter we will review the garlic supplements currently available. By the end of the chapter you'll know how much to take, and how to choose the most effective products for your particular needs.

Why We Need Supplements

If you want to take advantage of garlic's wide range of healing properties but are put off by the taste and smell of real garlic, supplements are the answer. They provide an opportunity to share in the unquestionable health benefits without experiencing any of the admittedly mild side effects.

As we've seen, garlic products have become extremely popular in the last few years, primarily in Northern Europe and in the United States, where garlic is not yet a national flavor. There are many garlic products on the market, from the comparatively odorous to the completely deodorized. These come in the form of oils, powders, extracts, pills, and capsules. How effective are they? Which ones are best? There has been a good deal of controversy in the marketplace in recent years about the advantages of different products. Many pseudoscientific statements have been made in the popular press by garlic supplement producers.

Garlic products can be divided into three main groups depending on how they are made. We'll look at the different types and discuss the pros and cons of each.

Dried Garlic Powder Tablets

This first and best type of supplement is the dried garlic tablet. These tablets are made by slicing garlic and then drying the slices in a specific way to preserve their potency. Garlic is nearly two-thirds water, so drying produces a powder that is then ready to put into tablets. These tablets can then be coated to reduce the aroma. This is a potentially good way of preserving the medicinal qualities of garlic, because it is possible to achieve high levels of allicin in such powders. They contain most of the alliin, the original active compound. When the tablets dissolve in the intestine, this alliin is converted to allicin, just as it is when fresh garlic is crushed. The good news is that the malodorous allicin is released far down in the digestive system, so that very little odor is expelled from the mouth. For this reason, these dried garlic tablets are often called "odor controlled." Garlic tablets have been subjected to many clinical trials, and they achieve nearly the same results as fresh garlic.

The garlic powder tablets are very popular, and most of the clinical trials on reducing cholesterol have used this kind of product.

The drying process sounds very simple, but is in fact very complicated. Special conditions are necessary in order to produce the maximum amounts of allicin and other active compounds in the dried powder.

Because there are the different methods for drying garlic, the powders can vary from very good to very poor. This variation presents a problem for the consumer, who has a right to know the potency of any product. Fortunately, there are two tests that can be performed to assess whether or not the powder contains high levels of allicin. One test is done in the laboratory by the manufacturer; the other is one that you can do yourself.

The Taste Test

This test you can do by yourself. Remember we said that allicin is pungent and burning, but it does not have a strong odor. The oily sulfides that are produced from allicin, on the other hand, have the typically rich, sulfurous aroma of garlic but do not have a burning taste. So, you can test the contents of a pill or capsule by taste. First, the taste should be strong. Second, it should have both the burning taste of allicin (the more the better) and the rich aroma of the sulfides.

The Laboratory Test

Responsible companies know that they have to guarantee the potency of the product. Therefore, they will analyze the powder and generally record the content on the label. Since allicin, the main active ingredient, may not be present in the tablet, but will be released in the intestine, the label may state "allicin," "allicin equivalent," or "allicin release." It is advisable to buy such "guaranteed potency" products that tell you specifically how much allicin they release.

If the powder is well made, it should be equally effective at protecting circulation, detoxifying the body, and fighting bacteria. Research to develop a highly effective garlic product is being actively pursued. In China, Europe, and the United States, efforts are being made to produce the perfect garlic powder extract for medicinal use.

Garlic Oil Capsules

Capsules containing garlic oil are the second best supplement on the market. Garlic oil is the essential or aromatic oil of garlic. It is made by mashing garlic in a vat and then bubbling steam through it. The oily components are carried through on the steam, and then collected once the steam has cooled.

Another way of making garlic oil is to add a large quantity of vegetable oil to mashed garlic in a vat, without heating it. The vegetable oil takes up the garlic oil, after which the solids are removed in filtration. This is called an oil macerate and is used to produce some European oil capsules.

The oil of garlic is made up of sulfides, disulfides, trisulfides, and other compounds that are formed from the transformation of allicin. In ordinary fresh garlic, or in fresh garlic mixed with vegetable oil, this change happens over a few days. When mashed garlic is steam distilled, it happens immediately because of the heat, as it does when garlic is fried. Garlic oil is therefore very similar to fried garlic. The amount of the oil is roughly the same as the amount of allicin that produced it, that is, 0.1 to 0.2 percent of the total weight. In other words, at least 500 to 1,000 kilograms of fresh garlic is needed to produce 1 kilogram of oil, making the oil extremely concentrated.

Garlic oil is normally sold in capsules, in which a very small amount is suspended in vegetable oil and enclosed in gelatin. These capsules were the very first garlic product, developed in the 1920s in Germany, and consistently popular ever since. In fact, most of the 300 million doses of garlic consumed in the United Kingdom in 1995 were in the form of garlic oil capsules.

Odor Controlled vs. Odorless
Garlic supplements are "odor controlled" if the active ingredients are released in the intestine, and "odorless" if the extract is not based on allicin or sulfides.

When you consume garlic capsules, you can avoid the mouth odor that comes from chewing garlic. How - ever, the contents of the capsules have a strong garlic odor that can emerge on the breath after the capsules are dissolved in the stomach. Manufacturers often reduce this odor even further by coating the capsules with a substance that prevents them from dissolving in the stomach. Instead, the capsules pass through it and dissolve in the intestine, thus avoiding the odor and burping that sometimes occurs with ordinary capsules.

How Effective Are Garlic Oil Capsules?

There have been a number of studies on this question. It has been found by scientists like Professor Arun Bordia, a pioneer of garlic research in India, and Dr. Asaf Qureshi, of the United States Department of Agriculture, that the oil is as effective as fresh garlic at reducing cholesterol and blood clotting, and as a general cardiovascular preventive. Thus, the popularity of garlic oil capsules over the years has been confirmed in the laboratory. However, the antibiotic potency of garlic oil capsules is limited. Studies have shown that fresh garlic or garlic juice that is placed in the middle of a "sea" of bacteria will kill all the bacteria within a distance of one to two inches. If garlic oil is used, the power to kill the bacteria or fungi is much reduced, though still present.

One clove of garlic will produce 2 to 6 milligrams of oil or 4 milligrams on average. As we shall see below, this is a minimum daily dose. Many capsules on the market today contain less than 1 milligram of oil, often only 0.66 milligrams. And therefore, one may need to consume four to six capsules per day (depending on their strength) to achieve the minimum preventive dose. This is the problem with many of the garlic oil products. In fact, a number of researchers, such as Dr. R. R. Samson of the Edinburgh Royal Infirmary, have carried out studies on patients using the oil capsules. In these studies, when oil that is freshly prepared in the laboratory is used, the thinning of the blood and the reducing of cholesterol can be clearly demonstrated. Unfortunately, when some oil capsules were used according to the manufacturer's recommendations, no results were obtained because the amount of garlic oil per capsule was insufficient. So, make sure that there is enough garlic in the capsules you are considering taking, and take enough to achieve a daily dose of at least 4 milligrams of garlic oil.

Deodorized "Aged" Garlic

The last garlic supplement to look at is deodorized garlic. You might encounter this product in health food stores. It is made by chopping garlic and aging it in alcohol over many months. An extract made from this substance is then used as the basis for tablets and other preparations. The process prevents the formation of allicin and the strong-smelling sulfides. The advantage, of course, is that the product does not smell at all. The disadvantage, however, is that the absence of allicin means that the product may be much less effective for some of the main beneficial uses of garlic. The aged garlic preparations therefore appear to have a rather different chemical profile from crushed garlic or other allicin-based garlic preparations.

There is quite a lot of debate in the health product industry and the scientific literature concerning the effectiveness of deodorized, as compared to regular, garlic products. The situation is unclear because there have never been clinical studies in which the effectiveness of different forms of garlic has been compared. The absence of such studies means that the debate is based on inference. Deodorized garlic appears to lack certain key ingredients that act on the circulation and have anti-infective effects, yet they have other ingredients that may have anticancer effects.

Though the different forms of garlic have not been compared clinically, the vast majority of clinical and scientific research on garlic powder tablets and garlic oil capsules shows that they are effective in heart protection and anti-infection, while the majority of studies on the aged deodorized garlic show that it may be effective as an aid in cancer prevention and as an agent in detoxification.

How Much Garlic to Take Daily?

Each manufacturer uses a different dose in preparation of the product, and different ways of preparing garlic lead to different concentrations of components. These differences create confusion. It would be wonderful if all the manufacturers could express their dosages as "equivalent to such-and-such number of grams of fresh garlic."

The correct daily dose of fresh garlic is between one and two cloves of garlic for cardiac health, and more for treating infections. This is given in the pharmacopoeias and the German Ministry of Health definitions. This is a minimum of about one-tenth of an ounce of fresh garlic per day. What is the correct dose of dried garlic tablets? Since fresh garlic is about two-thirds water, you will need to take a daily dose from 1 to 2 grams of tablets of dried garlic; for example, one to two tablets of 500 milligrams each morning and evening. The correct dose of concentrated extract or garlic oil varies depending on the brand. You will need a minimum of 4 milligrams of garlic oil per day, or extract, equivalent to 3 grams of fresh garlic. The package should clearly state what the correspondence is between a tablet or capsule and the equivalent amount of fresh garlic.

To figure out how many garlic supplements to

Quantities of Garlic

One clove of fresh garlic weighs about 3 grams. This is equivalent to 1 gram of dried garlic powder or 2 to 6 milligrams of garlic oil.

take, you need to know the correct dose of fresh garlic for comparison. Lets review the two levels of doses you should be aware of :

The "Preventive" Dose

For all preventive purposes, including the protection of circulation, you should take at least one clove of garlic, weighing from 2 to 3 grams, a day. This is the minimum dose—double this dose would be better. It is advisable to split the daily dose, as studies have shown that garlic stays in the body for just a few hours before it is removed or neutralized. Therefore, it is a good idea to take at least one to one and a half grams (or half a clove) in the morning and again in the evening.

The "Therapeutic" Dose

At times you will need to take much more than the preventive dose. If you are using garlic to treat an illness or a symptom, such as a bronchial or throat problem, Candida, stomach infections, skin infections, and so on, then a larger, therapeutic dose is required. The reason is that you need a much more powerful punch to knock out bacteria, yeast, or fungi than to inhibit cholesterol, fats, and blood clots in the circulation. However in more serious cases of circulatory disease or atherosclerosis, garlic may be used at a higher dose as part of a therapeutic program. The therapeutic dose should be a minimum of one clove's worth (2 to 3 grams) 3 times a day. This is the amount suggested by the British herbal pharmacopoeia, traditional sources, and modern herbal guides.

Safe and Effective

Garlic is absolutely safe. All over the world, garlic is consumed by millions of people daily without adverse effects. There are groups of people whose traditional foods include several cloves of fresh garlic daily, without any signs of harm. For example, the people of Guanshan County in Shandong

Province, China, consume about 20 grams of fresh garlic per day, that's about seven cloves. In some studies on cholesterol reduction, up to twenty cloves of fresh garlic per day were given for three months, without ill effects. People have taken 200 milligrams of garlic oil, the equivalent of seventy cloves of garlic, without ill effects.

Garlic is only toxic at excessively high doses. Studies in rats have shown that toxic effects occurred at a dose of 5 grams of fresh juice per kilogram (2.2 pounds) of body weight, which is equivalent to an average man eating 300 mashed cloves in one sitting. At this kind of dose, the stomach can be injured by the harshness of fresh garlic, as it would be by other biting substances such as red pepper.

Allicin itself, the pungent component in garlic, is also toxic at very high doses, beyond an amount that would ever be consumed people. In animal studies, liver and stomach toxicity occurred in rats that were given allicin at a dose equal to a man eating 500 cloves of garlic. Allicin or fresh garlic can cause a minor side effect if it is held against the skin or the delicate tissues of the mouth, where it can cause irritation or actual burning. In some people who are sensitive, handling a lot of garlic can cause skin rashes, an occasional prob-lem for professional cooks or workers in the food industry. The problem can be easily remedied by wearing latex gloves.

As mentioned in the chapter on garlic and the circulation, garlic can slow blood clotting. Although this is normally desirable for cardiovascular health, people who are taking anti-clotting drugs should be aware that garlic can further reduce the clot-ting tendency of the blood. In certain situations, such as during surgery, blood clotting should not be slowed. So, you shouldn't take garlic before a scheduled operation.

Some people occasionally experience heartburn, "burping," or some mild digestive discomfort. But this happens only after eating fresh garlic, not from consuming garlic supplements, and it passes rapidly. As previously mentioned, the smell of garlic is the main reason why some people avoid it. But medicines don't always taste or smell good, so this can hardly be called a "side effect."

In this chapter, you've seen that there are different ways of taking garlic supplements. But don't forget, there is nothing like fresh garlic—the best and cheapest way to take advantage of garlic's medicinal properties.

CONCLUSION

Now you know a great deal about garlic. From its important role in preventing and controlling different aspects of heart disease to that of helping to ease the discomfort of the common cold, garlic has been shown to be the archetypical natural remedy. So why not put this guide down, go out, and try garlic for yourself. If you have never tried natural remedies before, the whole concept of self-treatment and natural approaches might feel a bit daunting. It's worth remembering that before the advent of modern medicine (only about 100 years ago), people treated their illnesses, both major and minor, with an array of natural remedies, such as garlic. Modern medicine has made valuable and life-saving contributions to the world but, sadly, has also led to a dismissal of the vast amount of ancient knowledge of nature's gifts to our well-being. Many of these ancient prescriptions can be as effective in improving our lives as many modern medicines—and are often much safer. By returning to the healing solutions of our forefathers, we join the great continuum of traditional knowledge for self-care. So whether your first port of call is the kitchen or the health food store, be aware that you are following a long and wise tradition.

SELECTED REFERENCES

Adetumbi, M. A. and B. H. S. Lau. *Allium sativum* (gar - lic)—a natural antibiotic. *Medical Hypotheses*, 1983; 12: 227–237.

Belman, S. Onion and garlic oils and tumour promotion. *Carcinogenesis*, 1983; 4: 1063–1065.

Block, E. The chemistry of garlic and onions. *Scientific American*, 1985; 252: 94–97.

Boullin, D. J. Garlic as a platelet inhibitor, *Lancet*, 1983; 1: 776–777.

Caporaso, L., S. M. Smith, and R H. K. Eng. Antifungal activity in human urine and serum after ingestion of garlic (*Allium sativum*). *Antimicrobio. Agents Chemotherap*, 1983; 23: 700–702.

De Santos, O. S., and J. Grunwald. Effect of garlic powder tablets on blood lipids and blood pressure: A six month, placebo controlled, double-blind study. *British J. Clinical Research*, 1993; 4: 37–44.

Ernst, E., I. Weihmayr, and A. Matrai. Garlic and blood lipids. *British Medical Journal*, 1985; 291:139.

Fenwick, G. R. and A. B. Hanley. The Genus Allium, Parts 1–3. *Critical Reviews on Food Science*, 1986; Vols 22 and 23.

Fleischauer, A. T. Garlic consumption and cancer prevention: Meta-analyses of colorectal and stomach cancers. *American Journal of Clinical Nutrition*, 2000; 72: 1047–1052.

Jain, A. K., et al. Can garlic reduce levels of serum lipids? A controlled clinical study. *American Journal of Medicine*, 1993; 94: 632–635.

Jung, F., et al. Effect of different garlic preparations on the fluidity of blood, fibrinolytic activity, and peripheral microcirculation in comparison with placebo. *Planta Medica*, 1990; 56: 668.

Kennel, W. Cholesterol in the prediction of atherosclerotic disease: new perspective based on the Framingham study. *Annals of Internal Medicine*, 1979; 90:85.

Keyes, A. Wine, Garlic and CHD in seven countries. *Lancet*, 1980; 1:145–146.

Lawson, L.D. Bioactive organosulfur compounds of garlic and garlic products: Role in reducing blood lipids. In: *Human Medicinal Agents from Plants*, A. D. Kinghorn, and M. F. Balandrin, eds. 1993., Washington, D.C.: American Chemical Society Books.

Mader, F. H. Treatment of hyperlipidaemia with garlic-powder tablets. *Drug Research*, 1990; 40: 1111–1116.

Mirelman, D. Inhibition of growth of Entamoeba histolytica by allicin, the active principle of garlic extract. *J. Infectious Diseases*, 1987; 156: 243–244.

Moore, G. S. and R. D. Atkins. Fungicidal and fungi - static effects of an aqueous garlic extract on medically important yeast-like fungi. *Mycologia*, 1997; 69: 341–348.

Rees, L.P., et al. A quatitative assessment of the antimicrobial activity of garlic (Allium sativum). *World Journal of Microbiology and Biotechnology*, 1993; 9: 303–307.

Sainanl, B.S., et al. Effect of dietary garlic and onion on serum lipid profile in a Jain community. *Indian J. Med. Research*, 1979; 69: 776–780.

Silagy, C. and A. Neil. Garlic as a lipid-lowering agent: A meta-analysis. *Journal of the Royal College of Physicians*, 1994; 28: 39–45.

Stevinson, C., M. H. Pittler, and E. Ernst. Garlic for treating hypercholesterolemia. A meta-analysis of randomized clinical trials. *Annals of Internal Medicine* 2000; 133: 420–429.

Wargovich, M. J. Inhibition of gastrointestinal cancer by organosulfur compounds in garlic. *Cancer Chemoprevention*, 1992; 195–203.

Weisberger, H. S. and J. Pensky. Tumour-inhibiting effects derived from an active principle of garlic (*Allium sativum*) *Science*, 1957; 126: 1112–1114.

OTHER BOOKS
AND RESOURCES

Fulder, S. *The Garlic Book.* Garden City Park, NY: Avery, 1997.

Koch, H. P., and Lawson, L. D. *Garlic—The Science and Therapeutic Application of Allium sativum L. and Related Species.* Baltimore, MD: Williams and Wilkins, 1996.

GreatLife Magazine
Consumer magazine with articles on vitamins, minerals, herbs, and foods.
Available for free at many health and natural food stores.

Let's Live Magazine
Consumer magazine with emphasis on the health benefits of vitamins, minerals, and herbs.
Customer service:
1-800-676-4333
P.O. Box 74908
Los Angeles, CA 90004
Subscriptions: 12 issues per year, $19.95 in the U.S.; $31.95 outside the U.S.

The Nutrition Reporter™ newsletter
Monthly newsletter that summarizes recent medical research on vitamins, minerals, and herbs.
Customer service:
P.O. Box 30246
Tucson, AZ 85751-0246
e-mail: jack@thenutritionreporter.com
www.nutritionreporter.com
Subscriptions: 12 issues per year, $26 in the U.S.; $32 U.S. or $48 CNC for Canada; $38 for other countries.

INDEX

Academy of Medicine
Pediatric Institute,
43–44
Africa, 64
AIDS, 49
Ajoene, 56
Alcohol, 20–21
Allicin, 48, 49, 54–57,
76–78, 83
function, 56
Alliin, 53–54, 76
Allium sativum. See Garlic.
Amoebas, 49–50
Anginal pain, 25
*Annals of Internal
Medicine*, 17
Antibiotics, 42–51
Aristotle, 4, 65
Ascorbic acid. *See* Vitamin
C.
Atherosclerosis, 19, 25, 27,
30, 64
Atherosclerosis, 30
Athlete's foot, 46, 71
Ayurvedic medicine, 63, 66

Bacteria, 6–7, 42–51
Balms, 65
Barley, 9
Barone, Frank, 47
Beeton, Mrs., 61
Belman, Sydney, 39
Beta-carotene, 9
Bible, The, 59
Bile, 21
Block, Erick, 56
Blood cells, white, 43, 46, 49
Blood circulation, 1, 5, 7,
12, 27–30, 64. *See also*
Circulatory system.
Blood clots. *See*
Thromboses.
Blood pressure, 1, 29
Blood pressure, high, 1, 6,
24, 27–30
Blood sugar, 24

Blood thinners, 1, 5,
30–32, 83
Blood vessels, 1, 5
*Book of Household
Management*, 61
Bordia, Arun, 79
Boullin, Professor, 30
British Medical Journal, 33
Bronchitis, 7, 43–44, 70

*Canadian Journal of
Physiology and
Pharmacology*, 36
Cancer, 4, 6, 37–42
Candida albicans, 7,
46–48, 71
See also Yeast.
Caporaso, Neil, 48
Case Western Reserve
University, 38
Catarrh, 8, 44
Charaka, 63
Chest, 9
China, 39, 52, 66, 82–83
Chives, 52
Cholesterol, 1, 9, 12–22, 24
high-density (HDL),
15–16, 18, 20
low-density (LDL), 15–16,
18, 20
Cholesterol-lowering
drugs, 19
Cigarette smoke, 21, 24
Circulatory system, 5, 25,
70. *See also* Blood
circulation.
Cloves, oil, 9
Codex Ebers, 37
Colds, 7, 49
Companion planting, 74
Compost, 73
Coughs, 43
Cysteine, 37, 57
Cystitis, 46

Dairy products, 70

Degenerative diseases, 24
Detoxification, 35–41
Diabetes, 13
Diet, 13, 24. *See also* Food.
Dioscorides, 60, 63
Drug Research, 17, 28

Ebers Papyrus, 59
Edema, 63
Edinburgh Royal Infirmary, 79
Egyptians, ancient, 37, 58–59
Elizabeth I, Queen of England, 61
Ernst, E., 33
Estrogen, 12
Europe, Eastern, 42, 44, 45, 64, 65
Europe, medieval, 60–61
Evelyn, John, 61
Exercise, 13, 19, 24, 27

Fasting, 47
Fat, 5
Fats, 18
  hydrogenated, 24
  saturated, 13, 20, 24, 30
Fiber, 9, 13, 20–21
Finland, 14
First aid balms, 65
Fish oils, 9, 21
Food, 9
  medicinal, 9–11, 19
  processed, 35
  unprocessed, 21
  See also Diet.
Fungi, 6–7, 45–48, 71

Gaius Pliny, 60
Galen, 60
Gardening, 72–74
Garlic, 1–2, 3–11, 12–22, 23–34, 35–41, 42–51, 52–57, 58–66, 67–74, 75–84, 85
  basics, 52–57
  bulbs, 52–54
  cancer and, 37–41
  cautions, 50
  cholesterol and, 12–22
  cooking and, 67–72
  deodorized, 80–81

detoxification and, 34–41
dosages, 22, 33, 79, 81–83
external applications, 71
folk traditions, 62–66
forms, 71
gardening, 72–74
harvesting, 73–74
heart disease and, 23–34
history, 3, 58–66
how it works, 17–18
in milk, 70
in the kitchen, 67–72
infections and, 42–51
magic and mystery of, 65–66
medicinal ingredients, 53–54, 69–71
odor, 67, 72
oil capsules, 77–80
planting, 72–73
prejudice against, 61–62
recipes, 68–71
safety, 82–84
storage, 74
studies, 17–19, 26, 29, 30–31, 38–40, 44–45, 47–48
supplements, 75–84
suppositories, 49
syrup, 70
tablets, 76–77
Genetics, 13
George Washington University School of Medicine, 5, 31
German Health Ministry, 7, 81
Gilroy, C.A., 53
Glucose. *See* Blood sugar.
Greeks, ancient, 59–60, 65
Gypsies, 63

Health Ministry, Japan, 8
Heart, 2, 4–6, 23–34
Heart attacks, 5, 14–15, 25, 28
Heart disease, 4–7, 12, 14–15, 20, 23–34
  prevention, 33–34
  reversing, 32
  risk factors, 24
Heavy metals. *See* Metals, heavy.

Henry IV, King of France,
 60–61
Herbal Drugs Commission
 (E), Germany, 7
Herbalists, 66
Herbs, 9–11
High-density lipoprotein
 (HDL). *See* Cholesterol.
Hippocrates, 10, 59–60
Holistic medicine, 66
Hypertension. *See* Blood
 pressure, high.

Immune system, 38, 41, 43
India, 52, 63, 66
Infections, 4, 6–7, 42–51,
 64–65, 71
Iowa Women's Health
 Study, 39

Japan, 8, 14, 18, 26, 33
Jews, ancient, 59
*Journal of the American
 Medical Association,* 32
*Journal of the Royal
 College of Physicians,*
 29

Kidney failure, 28
Korea, 18
Kritchevsky, David, 17

Lancet, 3, 30, 31
Lead, 37
Leeks, 52
Leewenhoek, Anthony, 42
Lifestyle, 21–22, 32
Lipoproteins, 15
Liver, 13, 22, 36–37
Low-density lipoprotein
 (LDL). *See* Cholesterol.

Mader, F.H., 17
Magnesium, 24
Measure for Measure, 61
*Medical Journal of
 Australia,* 48
Mei, Xing, 39
Mercury, 37
Metals, heavy, 36–37
Ministry of Health, UK, 8
Mirelman, David, 49
Miso soup, 70–71

Mohammed, 65
Moscow Evening News, 44
Mouth infections, 71
Mucus, 44

National Cancer Institute,
 39
Natural killer (NK) cells, 43
Nebraska Medical Center, 9
New Jersey Medical
 University, 48
New York Medical Center,
 39
New York Times, 9
Nobel Prize, 55
Nutrition. *See* Diet.

Oats, 9
Obesity, 13, 24
Oil capsules, 77–80
Oil macerate, 78
Onions, 31, 52, 57
Ornish, Dean, 32–33

Panacea, 3–4
Parasites, 49
Pasteur, Louis, 44
Peripheral vascular
 disease, 30
Pharmacopoeia, 70
Pinworms, 49
Platelets, 25
Pollution, 35–36
Proteus, 44

Qureshi, Asaf, 79

Rabindranath Tagore Med -
 ical College Cardiology
 Dept., India, 18
Ratinsky, T., 44
Rees, Dr., 45
Rennard, Stephen, 9
Rhinitis, 8
Ringworm, 46, 48
Romans, 59–60, 65
Russia, 27, 42, 44, 45, 63

Sainani, Dr., 26
Salmonella, 44–45
Samson, R.R., 79
Sassoon General Hospital,
 26

Satal, 37
Schweitzer, Albert, 64
Scientific American, 3, 56
Sclerosis, 25
Selenium, 53
Seventh Day Adventists,
    19–20
Shakespeare, 61
Shallots, 52
Shandong Medical
    College, 39
Shigella, 44
Sinusitis, 7
Skin, 7, 71
Soil, 73–74
Soy, 70–71
Spain, 8, 52
Spices, 10, 71
State University of New
    York–Albany, 31, 56
Steinmetz, K., 39
Stress, 13, 19, 21–22, 24, 32
Strokes, 2, 5, 25, 28, 30
Sugar, 20–21. *See also*
    Blood sugar.
Sulfides, 55
Sulfur, 36–37, 40, 49, 53, 55
Supplements, 75–84
    deodorized, 78–81
    laboratory test, 77
    odor controlled versus
        odorless, 78–79
    oil capsules, 77–80
    tablets, 76–77
    taste test, 77
Suppositories, 49
Switzerland, 8

Tansey, Michael, 47
Tea, green, 9
Testosterone, 12
Threadworms, 49
Throats, sore, 7, 9
Thromboses, 25, 30–32
Thrush, 46
Thyme, 9
Toxins, 6, 35–41
Traditional medicine, 64–65
Trojan War, 59
Tuburculosis, 50
Turner, William, 61, 63
Tutankhamen, 4, 42, 58–59

United Kingdom, 8
United Nations, 52
University of California–
    Davis, 45
University of Delaware, 31
University of Indiana, 47, 55
University of Londrina, 44
University of Munich, 33
University of Texas, 40
University of Utah, 31
University of Western
    Ontario, 26
U.S. Department of
    Agriculture, 17, 18, 79
    Reasearch Laboratories,
    18, 55
U.S. National Institutes of
    Health, 14, 16

Vaginal yeast infections, 46
Vampires, 65
Vegetables, 9, 21
Vegetarians, 20, 21, 68
Veterans Administration
    Medical Center, 48
Victorians, 61–62
Viruses, 48–51
Vitaanen, Artur, 55
Vitamin B complex, 24, 53
Vitamin C, 21, 24, 53
Vitamin E, 21, 24, 53
Vitamins, 24

Walking, 27
Wargovich, Michael, 40
Weight, 21
Weissberger, A.S., 38
Weizmann Institute, 38, 49
Winthrop Chemical
    Company, 54
Wistar Institute,
    Philadelphia, 17
World Health
    Organization, 14
*World Journal of
    Microbiology and
    Biotechnology*, 45
World War I, 64
World War II, 64, 67
Worms, 49

Yeast, 45–51